MW00451394

Sirtfood Diet

The star's secret weapon diet, lose weight by eating super foods with a ready-to-use 21-day diet plan and quick and easy recipes

Michelle Prescott

Table of contents

INTRODUCTION

Trendy new diets seem to pop up regularly, and the Sirtfood Diet is one of the latest.

You might have heard of the Sirtfood Plan before - especially since it was reported singer Adele lost 50lbs following the plan - but do you know what it actually is?

It has become a favorite of celebrities in Europe and is famous for allowing red wine and chocolate. Its creators insist that it's not a fad, but rather that "sirtfoods" are the secret to unlocking fat loss and preventing disease.

"Sirtfood" sounds like something developed by aliens, brought to earth for human consumption in the hopes of gaining mind control and world domination. In actuality, sirtfoods are simply foods high in sirtuins. Uh, come again? Sirtuins are a type of protein that studies on fruit flies and mice have shown regulate metabolism, increase muscle mass, and burn fat.

The plan in the book can help you burn fat and boost your energy, priming your body for long-term weight-loss success and a longer, healthier, disease-free life. All that while drinking red wine. Sounds like pretty much the perfect diet, right? Well, before you burn through your savings stocking up on sirtuins-filled ingredients, read the pros and cons.

The eating plan will change the way you do healthy eating. It may sound like a non-user-friendly name, but it's one you'll be hearing about a lot.

Because the 'Sirt' in Sirtfoods is shorthand for the sirtuin genes, a group of genes nicknamed the 'skinny genes' that work, frankly, like magic.

However, health experts warn that this diet may not live up to the hype and could even be a bad idea.

The eating plan defines the foods that turn on your so-called 'skinny genes', boosting your metabolism and your energy levels. In fact, it stipulates that you could lose 7lbs in 7 days...

According to the diet's founders, these special foods work by activating specific proteins in the body called sirtuins.

These foods contain high levels of plant chemicals called polyphenols, which are thought to switch on the Sirtuin genes and so provoke their super-healthy benefits.

Sirtuins are believed to protect cells in the body from dying when they are under stress and are thought to regulate inflammation, metabolism, and the aging process. It's thought that sirtuins influence the body's ability to burn fat and boost metabolism, resulting in a seven pound weight loss a week while maintaining muscle. However, some experts believe this is unlikely to be solely fat loss, but will instead reflect changes in glycogen stores from skeletal muscle and the liver.

Eating these foods, say the creators of the plan, nutritionists Aidan Goggins and Glen Matten, turn on these genes and "mimics the effects of calorie restriction, fasting, and exercise". It activates a recycling process in the body, "that clears out the cellular debris and clutter which accumulates over time and causes ill health and loss of vitality," write the authors.

The top Sirtfoods include red wine, cocoa (dark chocolate!), and coffee. Buckwheat is the main carb on the list, and such was the success of the first book – The Sirtfood Diet – when it launched last year, that health food shops sold out of it, and buckwheat noodle manufacturer Clearspring had to double its production.

HOW EFFECTIVE?

So far, there's no convincing evidence that the Sirtfood Diet has a more beneficial effect on weight loss than any other calorie-restricted diet.

And although many of these foods have healthful properties, there have not been any long-term human studies to determine whether eating a diet rich in sirtfoods has any tangible health benefits.

Nevertheless, the Sirtfood Diet book reports the results of a pilot study conducted by the authors and involving 39 participants from their fitness center. However, the results of this study appear not to have been published anywhere else.

For one week, the participants followed the diet and exercised daily. At the end of the week, participants lost an average of 7 pounds (3.2 kg) and maintained or even gained muscle mass.

Yet these results are hardly surprising. Restricting your calorie intake to 1,000 calories and exercising at the same time will nearly always cause weight loss.

Regardless, this kind of quick weight loss is neither genuine nor long-lasting, and this study did not follow participants after the first week to see if they gained any of the weight back, which is typically the case.

When your body is energy deprived, it uses up its emergency energy stores, or glycogen, in addition to burning fat and muscle.

Each molecule of glycogen requires 3–4 molecules of water to be stored. When your body uses up glycogen, it gets rid of this water as well. It's known as "water weight."

In the first week of extreme calorie restriction, only about one-third of the weight loss comes from fat, while the other two-thirds come from water, muscle, and glycogen.

As soon as your calorie intake increases, your body replenishes its glycogen stores, and the weight comes right back.

Unfortunately, this type of calorie restriction can also cause your body to lower its metabolic rate, causing you to need even fewer calories per day for energy than before.

It is likely that this diet may help you lose a few pounds in the beginning, but it will likely come back as soon as the diet is over.

As far as preventing disease, three weeks is probably not long enough to have any measurable long-term impact.

On the other hand, adding sirtfoods to your regular diet over the long-term may very well be a good idea. But in that case, you might as well skip the diet and start doing that now.

FOLLOWING THE SIRTFOOD DIET

The Sirtfood Diet has two phases that last a total of three weeks. After that, you can continue "sirtifying" your diet by including as many sirtfoods as possible in your meals.

Most of the ingredients and sirtfoods are easy to find.

However, three of the signature ingredients required for these two phases — matcha green tea powder, lovage, and buckwheat — may be expensive or difficult to find.

A big part of the diet is its green juice, which you'll need to make yourself between one and three times daily. You will need a juicer (a blender will not work) and a kitchen scale, as the ingredients are listed by weight. The recipe is below:

Sirtfood Green Juice

75 grams (2.5 oz) kale

30 grams (1 oz) arugula (rocket)

5 grams parsley

2 celery sticks

1 cm (0.5 in) ginger

half a green apple

half a lemon

half a teaspoon matcha green tea

Juice all ingredients except for the green tea powder and lemon together, and pour them into a glass. Juice the lemon by hand, then stir both the lemon juice and green tea powder into your juice.

Phase One

The first phase lasts seven days and involves calorie restriction and lots of green juice. It is intended to jump-start your weight loss and claimed to help you lose 7 pounds (3.2 kg) in seven days.

During the first three days of phase one, calorie intake is restricted to 1,000 calories. You drink three green juices per day plus one meal. Each day you can choose from recipes in the book, which all involve sirtfoods as a main part of the meal.

Meal examples include miso-glazed tofu, the sirtfood omelet, or a shrimp stir-fry with buckwheat noodles.

On days 4–7 of phase one, calorie intake is increased to 1,500. This includes two green juices per day and two more sirtfood-rich meals, which you can choose from the book.

Phase Two

Phase two lasts for two weeks. During this "maintenance" phase, you should continue to steadily lose weight.

There is no specific calorie limit for this phase. Instead, you eat three meals full of sirtfoods and one green juice per day. Again, the meals are chosen from recipes provided in the book.

After the Diet

You may repeat these two phases as often as desired for further weight loss.

However, you are encouraged to continue "sirtifying" your diet after completing these phases by incorporating sirtfoods regularly into your meals.

There are a variety of Sirtfood Diet books that are full of recipes rich in sirtfoods. You can also include sirtfoods in your diet as a snack or in recipes you already use.

Additionally, you are encouraged to continue drinking the green juice every day.

In this way, the Sirtfood Diet becomes more of a lifestyle change than a one-time diet.

THE NEW SUPERFOODS

There's no denying that sirtfoods are good for you. They are often high in nutrients and full of healthy plant compounds.

Moreover, studies have associated many of the foods recommended on the Sirtfood Diet with health benefits.

For example, eating moderate amounts of dark chocolate with a high cocoa content may lower the risk of heart disease and help fight inflammation.

Drinking green tea may reduce the risk of stroke and diabetes and help lower blood pressure.

And turmeric has anti-inflammatory properties that have beneficial effects on the body in general and may even protect against chronic, inflammation-related diseases.

In fact, the majority of sirtfoods have demonstrated health benefits in humans.

However, evidence on the health benefits of increasing sirtuin protein levels is preliminary. Yet, research in animals and cell lines have shown exciting results.

For example, researchers have found that increased levels of certain sirtuin proteins lead to a longer lifespan in yeast, worms, and mice.

And during fasting or calorie restriction, sirtuin proteins tell the body to burn more fat for energy and improve insulin sensitivity. One study in mice found that increased sirtuin levels led to fat loss.

Some evidence suggests that sirtuins may also play a role in reducing inflammation, inhibiting the development of tumors, and slowing the development of heart disease and Alzheimer's.

While studies in mice and human cell lines have shown positive results, there have been no human studies examining the effects of increasing sirtuin levels.

Therefore, whether increasing sirtuin protein levels in the body will lead to the longer lifespan or a lower risk of cancer in humans is unknown.

Research is currently underway to develop compounds effective at increasing sirtuin levels in the body. This way, human studies can begin to examine the effects of sirtuins on human health.

Until then, it's not possible to determine the effects of increased sirtuin levels.

IS IT SUSTAINABLE?

Sirtfoods are almost all healthy choices and may even result in some health benefits due to their antioxidant or anti-inflammatory properties.

Yet eating just a handful of particularly healthy foods cannot meet all of your body's nutritional needs.

The Sirtfood Diet is unnecessarily restrictive and offers no clear, unique health benefits over any other type of diet.

Furthermore, eating only 1,000 calories is typically not recommended without the supervision of a physician. Even eating 1,500 calories per day is excessively restrictive for many people.

The diet also requires drinking up to three green juices per day. Although juices can be a good source of vitamins and minerals, they are also a source of sugar and contain almost none of the healthy fiber that whole fruits and vegetables do.

What's more, sipping on juice throughout the whole day is a bad idea for both your blood sugar and your teeth.

Not to mention, because the diet is so limited in calories and food choice, it is more than likely deficient in protein, vitamins, and minerals, especially during the first phase.

Due to the low calorie levels and restrictive food choices, this diet may be difficult to stick to for the entire three weeks.

Add that to the high initial costs of having to purchase a juicer, the book, and certain rare and expensive ingredients, as well as the time costs of preparing specific meals and juices, and this diet becomes unfeasible and unsustainable for many people.

The Bottom Line

The Sirtfood Diet is full of healthy foods, but not healthy eating patterns.

Not to mention, its theory and health claims are based on grand extrapolations from preliminary scientific evidence.

While adding some sirtfoods to your diet is not a bad idea and may even offer some health benefits, the diet itself looks like just another fad.

Save yourself the money and skip to making healthful, long-term dietary changes instead.

SO WHAT IS IT ALL ABOUT?

Two celebrity nutritionists working for a private gym in the UK developed the Sirtfood Diet.

They advertise the diet as a revolutionary new diet and health plan that works by turning on your "skinny gene."

This diet is based on research on sirtuins (SIRTs), a group of seven proteins found in the body that has been shown to regulate a variety of functions, including metabolism, inflammation, and lifespan.

Certain natural plant compounds may be able to increase the level of these proteins in the body, and foods containing them have been dubbed "sirtfoods."

So what are these magical 'sirtfoods'? The list of the "top 20 sirtfoods" provided by the Sirtfood Diet includes:

KALE
Of all the super healthy greens, kale is king. It is definitely one of the healthiest and most nutritious plant foods in existence. Kale is loaded with all sorts of beneficial compounds, some of which have powerful medicinal properties.

Here are 10 health benefits of kale that are supported by science.

1. Kale Is Among The Most Nutrient-Dense Foods on The Planet

Kale is a popular vegetable and a member of the cabbage family.

It is a cruciferous vegetable like cabbage, broccoli, cauliflower, collard greens, and Brussels sprouts.

There are many different types of kale. The leaves can be green or purple and have either a smooth or curly shape.

The most common type of kale is called curly kale or Scots kale, which has green and curly leaves and a hard, fibrous stem.

A single cup of raw kale (about 67 grams or 2.4 ounces) contains (1):

Vitamin A: 206% of the DV (from beta-carotene)

Vitamin K: 684% of the DV

Vitamin C: 134% of the DV

Vitamin B6: 9% of the DV

Manganese: 26% of the DV

Calcium: 9% of the DV

Copper: 10% of the DV

Potassium: 9% of the DV

Magnesium: 6% of the DV

It also contains 3% or more of the DV for vitamin B1 (thiamin), vitamin B2 (riboflavin), vitamin B3 (niacin), iron and phosphorus

This is coming with a total of 33 calories, 6 grams of carbs (2 of which are fiber), and 3 grams of protein.

Kale contains very little fat, but a large portion of the fat in it is an omega-3 fatty acid called alpha-linolenic acid.

Given its incredibly low-calorie content, kale is among the most nutrient-dense foods in existence. Eating more kale is a great way to dramatically increase the total nutrient content of your diet.

Kale is very high in nutrients and very low in calories, making it one of the most nutrient-dense foods on the planet.

2. Kale Is Loaded With Powerful Antioxidants Like Quercetin and Kaempferol

Kale, like other leafy greens, is very high in antioxidants.

These include beta-carotene and vitamin C, as well as various flavonoids and polyphenols.

Antioxidants are substances that help counteract oxidative damage by free radicals in the body.

Oxidative damage is believed to be among the leading drivers of aging and many diseases, including cancer.

But many substances that happen to be antioxidants also have other important functions.

This includes the flavonoids quercetin and kaempferol, which are found in relatively large amounts in kale.

These substances have been studied thoroughly in test tubes and animals.

They have powerful heart-protective, blood pressure-lowering, anti-inflammatory, anti-viral, anti-depressant, and anti-cancer effects, to name a few.

3. It Is an Excellent Source of Vitamin C

Vitamin C is an important water-soluble antioxidant that serves many vital functions in the body's cells.

For example, it is necessary for the synthesis of collagen, the most abundant structural protein in the body.

Kale is much higher in vitamin C than most other vegetables, containing about 4.5 times much as spinach.

The truth is, kale is actually one of the world's best sources of vitamin C. A cup of raw kale contains even more vitamin C than a whole orange.

4. Kale Can Help Lower Cholesterol, Which May Reduce The Risk of Heart Disease

Cholesterol has many important functions in the body.

For instance, it is used to make bile acids, which is are substances that help the body digest fats.

The liver turns cholesterol into bile acids, which are then released into the digestive system whenever you eat a fatty meal.

When all the fat has been absorbed and the bile acids have served their purpose, they are reabsorbed into the bloodstream and used again.

Substances called bile acid sequestrants can bind bile acids in the digestive system and prevent them from being reabsorbed. This reduces the total amount of cholesterol in the body.

Kale actually contains bile acid sequestrants, which can lower cholesterol levels. This might lead to a reduced risk of heart disease over time.

One study found that drinking kale juice every day for 12 weeks increased HDL (the "good") cholesterol by 27% and lowered LDL levels by 10%, while also improving antioxidant status.

According to one study, steaming kale dramatically increases the bile acid binding effect. Steamed kale is actually 43% as potent as cholestyramine, a cholesterol-lowering drug that functions in a similar way.

5. Kale Is One of The World's Best Sources of Vitamin K

Vitamin K is an important nutrient.

It is absolutely critical for blood clotting and does this by "activating" certain proteins and giving them the ability to bind calcium.

The well-known anticoagulant drug Warfarin actually works by blocking the function of this vitamin.

Kale is one of the world's best sources of vitamin K, with a single raw cup containing almost 7 times the recommended daily amount.

The form of vitamin K in kale is K1, which is different than vitamin K2. K2 is found in fermented soy foods and certain animal products. It helps prevent heart disease and osteoporosis.

6. There Are Numerous Cancer-Fighting Substances in Kale

Cancer is a terrible disease characterized by the uncontrolled growth of cells.

Kale is actually loaded with compounds that are believed to have protective effects against cancer.

One of these is sulforaphane, a substance that has been shown to help fight the formation of cancer at the molecular level.

It also contains an indole-3-carbinol, another substance that is believed to help prevent cancer.

Studies have shown that cruciferous vegetables (including kale) may significantly lower the risk of several cancers, although the evidence in humans is mixed.

7. Kale Is Very High in Beta-Carotene

Kale is often claimed to be high in vitamin A, but this is not entirely accurate.

It is actually high in beta-carotene, an antioxidant that the body can turn into vitamin A.

For this reason, kale can be an effective way to increase your body's levels of this very important vitamin.

8. Kale Is a Good Source of Minerals That Most People Don't Get Enough Of

Kale is high in minerals, some of which many people are deficient in.

It is a good plant-based source of calcium, a nutrient that is very important for bone health and plays a role in all sorts of cellular functions.

It is also a decent source of magnesium, an incredibly important mineral that most people don't get enough of. Eating plenty of magnesium may be protective against type 2 diabetes and heart disease.

Kale also contains quite a bit of potassium, a mineral that helps maintain electrical gradients in the body's cells. Adequate potassium intake has been linked to reduced blood pressure and a lower risk of heart disease.

One advantage that kale has over leafy greens like spinach is that it is low in oxalate, a substance found in some plants that can prevent minerals from being absorbed.

9. Kale Is High in Lutein and Zeaxanthin, Powerful Nutrients That Protect the Eyes

One of the most common consequences of aging is that eyesight gets worse.

Fortunately, there are several nutrients in the diet that can help prevent this from happening.

Two of the main ones are lutein and zeaxanthin, carotenoid antioxidants that are found in large amounts in kale, and some other foods.

Many studies have shown that people who eat enough lutein and zeaxanthin have a much lower risk of macular degeneration and cataracts, two very common eye disorders.

10. Kale Should Be Able to Help You Lose Weight

Kale has several properties that make it a weight loss friendly food.

It is very low in calories but still provides significant bulk that should help you feel full.

Because of the low calorie and high water content, kale has a low energy density. Eating plenty of foods with a low energy density has been shown to aid weight loss in numerous studies.

Kale also contains small amounts of protein and fiber. These are two of the most important nutrients when it comes to losing weight.

Although there is no study directly testing the effects of kale on weight loss, it makes sense that it could be a useful addition to a weight loss diet.

The Bottom Line

Fortunately, adding kale to your diet is relatively simple. You can simply add it to your salads or use them in recipes.

A popular snack is kale chips, where you drizzle some extra virgin olive oil or avocado oil on your kale, add some salt, and then bake in it an oven until dry.

It tastes absolutely delicious and makes a great crunchy, super healthy snack.

A lot of people also add kale to their smoothies in order to boost their nutritional value.

At the end of the day, kale is definitely one of the healthiest and most nutritious foods on the planet.

If you want to dramatically boost the number of nutrients you take in, consider loading up on kale.

RED WINE

The health benefits of red wine have been debated for some time.

Many believe that a glass each day is a valuable part of a healthy diet, while others think wine is somewhat overrated.

Studies have repeatedly shown that moderate red wine consumption seems to lower the risk of several diseases, including heart disease.

However, there is a fine line between moderate and excessive intake.

Winding down with a glass of wine isn't too unusual to do after a long day at work, and now science claims that drinking a glass of wine at night is actually healthy for you. In fact, scientists claim that drinking red wine before bed can help you lose weight. Bring out the wine glasses and put on your comfiest PJs, this weight loss tip is almost too good to be true.

The study, which was published in 2015 by Washington State University, illustrates that a little bit of red wine before bed can actually help you in losing weight. According to Woman's Day, a compound called resveratrol is responsible for helping you shed the pounds. Resveratrol has been shown to convert "white fat" into "beige fat". Beige fat is a little bit easier to burn off, making it easier to get down to your goal body weight.

Another study, which was conducted by Harvard, found that weight loss and wine go hand-in-hand.

Researchers looked at the data between 20,000 women over a range of 13 years and concluded that those who drank two glasses of wine a day were 70% less likely to be overweight.

Why at night? A previous study in 2012 showed that when bees ate a diet supplemented with resveratrol they ate less and they lived longer than the bees who ate a normal diet. While we are not saying humans and bees are exactly alike, we'll take anything that lets us drink a few glasses of red wine with dinner without guilt.

The health experts at the Mayo Clinic also agree that resveratrol, found in a glass of red wine, is great for your heart as well. It helps prevent damage to your blood vessels, prevents blood clots, and can reduce bad cholesterol. And a study in France concluded resveratrol was actually able to slow down the production of cancerous cells.

While there are many health benefits of red wine, it also needs to be said that since it is alcohol, it should be consumed in moderation. Drinking more than two glasses of wine a night could cause weight gain, instead of losing it, due to the excess calories.

Thankfully, red wine isn't the only place you can find resveratrol. Blueberries, strawberries, and grapes are all natural sources. Make yourself a berry sangria and you are in business!

STRAWBERRIES

It is a hybrid of two wild strawberry species from North America and Chile. Strawberries are bright red, juicy, and sweet. They're an excellent source of vitamin C and manganese and also contain decent amounts of folate (vitamin B9) and potassium.

Strawberries have a very low sugar content. They contain just one teaspoon of sugar per 100 kg. In addition, they have pronounced effects on improving how the body handles sugary carbohydrates. What researchers have found is that if we add strawberries to sugary carbs it has the effect of reducing insulin demand. This has the effect of turning strawberries into a sustained energy releaser. Strawberries are therefore a significant Sirtfood for weight loss and a healthy long-term diet.

Strawberries are included in the top Sirtfoods as they are a notable source of the sirtuin activator fisetin.

Strawberries offer an astonishing 129 percent of the daily requirements of vitamin C, a known infection fighter. They are also packed with manganese and folate, as well as potassium with its co-factoring enzyme, superoxide dismutase. Low in calories and fats, strawberries are a rich source of anthocyanins, ellagitannins, flavonols, terpenoids, and phenolic and ellagic acids, all phytonutrients which together multiply anti-inflammatory potential. Minerals like copper for the healthy development of red blood cells are in abundance, as are fluoride, iron, and iodine.

Besides being anti-cancer, strawberries also contain potential neurological disease-fighting and anti-aging compounds. What's more, the free radical-zapping antioxidant activity is outstanding in strawberries, as are their blood glucose-leveling abilities.

However, consume strawberries in moderation because they still contain fructose, which may be harmful to your health in excessive amounts.

Strawberries are one of those unique fruits requiring no embellishment to make them one of the world's most sought-after plant-based foods and one of the top-20 Sirtfoods.

Strawberries are very rich in antioxidants and plant compounds, which may have benefits for heart health and blood sugar control. Usually consumed raw and fresh, these berries can also be used in a variety of jams, jellies, and desserts.

Nutrition facts

Strawberries mainly consist of water (91%) and carbohydrates (7.7%). They contain only minor amounts of fat (0.3%) and protein (0.7%).

Strawberries are an excellent addition to a healthy diet.

ONIONS

Onions are one of the most popular vegetables worldwide. While most children dislike their pungent and bitey flavor, most adults embrace and use them regularly. Red onions contain twice as many antioxidants as any other form of onion making them a powerful part of an anti-inflammatory diet and Sirtfood lifestyle. Red onions are one of the top 20 Sirtfoods.

Red onions are also a rich source of the flavonoid antioxidant and major sirtuin-activating nutrient quercetin and the polyphenol antioxidant anthocyanin. These antioxidants prevent the oxidation of dietary and cellular fatty acids. They are very powerful free radical scavengers that neutralize cancer cell growth and dramatically reduce whole body inflammation.

The anti-oxidant flavonoids are extremely rich in the outer layers of the onion. Many people will peel off the first few layers and lose much of these critical nutrients. Be sure to utilize the outer, fleshy edible portions as much as possible.

How Many Red Onions to Eat?

Simmering onions in a soup or broth will damage some of the anthocyanins but not the sirtuin-activating quercetin. The quercetin moves into the soup or broth. The lower the heat the more nutrients will be contained in the soup or broth. Studies have shown that 4-7 servings of red onions each week (equivalent to about

2-3 onions) have been associated with the greatest benefit in reducing colorectal, oral, laryngeal, esophageal & ovarian cancer.

Red onions should be stored in a cool, dry area with good airflow.

Until they are opened they should not be stored in a refrigerator or plastic bag as both of these have been shown to speed up spoilage. Once opened, it is best to store in refrigeration. Avoid any onions that are wet, soft, bruised, or have dark spots or mold on them.

Frequently Asked Questions With Red Onions

1. Do I Need to Purchase Organic Onions?

Because onions are covered in a thin skin and are very sharp and pungent they repel pests. They are not highly sprayed with toxic herbicides and pesticides and therefore can be purchased non-organic without significant risk from toxic chemical exposure.

2. How Do I Reduce the Effect Onions Have on My Breath?

You can reduce the negative effects onions and other sulfur-rich foods (garlic, shallots, radishes) have on your breath by consuming green veggies, bitter herbs such as dandelion, parsley, or cilantro and herbs such as rosemary, fennel and peppermint.

We often advise people to consume another Sirtfood, parsley, or make a green Sirtfood juice on days when you are consuming a lot of raw onion.

3. Do I Get the Same Benefits from Cooked Onions as I Do with Raw Onions?

No, you will certainly lose much of the nutrient content but you will still get some of the benefits so it is better to consume cooked onions than no onions at all.

5. Soy

Soy or soya milk is basically a plant milk, which is made by soaking dried soybeans and grinding them in water.

Soy milk is a hit amongst vegans who keep away from using any animal-based products. Talking about the nutritive properties, soy milk is an excellent source of high-quality proteins, isoflavones--which help in reducing bad cholesterol and provide you with vitamins.

The milk is free of the milk sugar (lactose) and is a good choice for people who are lactose intolerant. Also, it is a good alternative for those who are allergic to the protein content that is present in the cow's milk and is extremely good with weight-watchers.

Now you must be wondering how soy milk is better than cow's milk. Here are 5 benefits which will clear your doubt.

1. Soy milk reduces cholesterol: According to the Food and Drug Administration (FDA) of the US, soy protein as part of a diet low in saturated fat and cholesterol may significantly reduce the risk of coronary heart diseases.

Whereas the saturated fats found in cow's milk are unhealthy and can increase your cholesterol.

2.   Soy milk does not cause insulin dependent diabetes: According to Soya.be, although no general consensus exists among scientists, some studies have shown an association between drinking cow's milk in early life and the development of insulin dependent diabetes. This association does not exist with soy milk. Yay!

3.   Soy milk is rich in isoflavones: Soy milk contains isoflavones, which is the most important and unique content found in the milk. They are known to have many benefits including reduction of cholesterol, easing of menopause symptoms, prevention of osteoporosis, and reduction of risk for certain cancers. Cow's milk does not contain isoflavones (prostate cancer and breast cancer). Isoflavones are also antioxidants that protect our cells and DNA against oxidation.

4. Good for weight-loss: The most apparent advantage of soy milk over cow's milk in terms of weight-loss is the reduction in calories and sugar content. Unlike milk fat which is highly saturated and prone to form deposits, soy fat is good for weight-watchers. You can drink full fat soy milk or eat snacks or desserts made with soy milk without feeling guilty.

5.   Soy milk contains only vegetable proteins: Vegetable proteins cause less loss of calcium through the kidneys. It is known that a diet rich in animal and dairy protein creates a higher risk for osteoporosis. Vegetable proteins lower the intake of dietary cholesterol and unhealthy saturated fats.

6. Parsley

Some diet plans specify drinking parsley tea with a least one meal a day, leaving the would-be dieter to wonder how exactly parsley helps you drop the pounds. Unfortunately, parsley tea isn't a magic brew for dieters. Its mild diuretic properties can, however, help to jump-start your diet and boost your confidence as you lose water weight. Exercise and balanced meals are the surest paths to sensible weight loss. Always check with your doctor to plan the best weight-loss approach.

Theory

Parsley tea temporarily facilitates weight loss by helping the body rid itself of excess water. Water retention can be related to premenstrual syndrome, to excess sodium in your diet, to pregnancy, or to certain medications. Diuretic vegetables and teas help to flush the system of some of this excess fluid, according to the University of Maryland Medical Center. Although parsley tea is considered a mild diuretic, ask your health-care practitioner before trying it on your own. Do not drink it if you are taking prescription diuretics.

Additional Benefits

For people cutting calories, vegetable broths and teas provide additional nutrients that they may be forgoing as they avoid certain foods. Parsley contains high amounts of potassium and vitamin A, as well as folate, calcium, vitamin C, and phosphorus. It also contains a flavonoid known as quercetin. According to the University of Maryland Medical Center, quercetin's antioxidant properties may help to lower cholesterol and high blood pressure while protecting you from heart disease and certain cancers. It may also help to relieve symptoms of allergies.

Basic Recipe

If your health food store stocks parsley tea, use one teabag per cup of water up to three times a day. Otherwise, the dried parsley found in the grocer's aisle works just as well. Pour 1 cup boiling water over 2 teaspoons of dried parsley, steep for 10 minutes and strain.

Multi-Herb Tea

Herbalist Jeanne Rose suggests blending parsley with smaller portions of some other herbs known for their diuretic and cleansing properties. To use fresh herbs, pour 1 quart boiling water over 1 large bunch parsley, 1 chopped blackberry leaf, 1 chopped dandelion leaf, 10 cherry stems, and 1/2 teaspoon of celery tops, couch grass, corn silk, and fennel seed. Strain and drink the tea throughout the day. To use dried herbs, use three parts parsley to one part each of the herbs named in the fresh herbs recipe. Rose recommends drinking several cups of the tea for at least one day.

Considerations

Whatever merits other herbal weight loss remedies may -- or may not -- possess, parsley tea shouldn't be confused with supplements like hoodia. Manufacturers claim that the botanical hoodia suppresses appetite, which results in weight loss. Parsley tea, on the other hand, helps you lose inches only if that extra bulk comes from retained water. Additionally, even herbal diuretic teas can be dangerous if you also take prescription diuretics. Talk to a doctor before using herbal teas for any medical condition.

7. EXTRA VIRGIN OLIVE OIL

One of the most effective ways you can stave off the aging effects of time is to eat plenty of foods known as 'Sirtfoods'. That's because these foods have the ability to activate sirtuins – genes that keep us young and slim by instructing the body to repair and rejuvenate our cells.

Twenty foods have been identified as being top sirtuin-triggers, and Extra Virgin Olive Oil, or EVOO, comes up seventh on the list. This is thanks to olives' content of two nutrients, in particular, oleuropein and hydroxytyrosol. These antioxidant polyphenols help keep the plants healthy, hardy, and resistant to disease – and when we eat them, we get those same benefits. Studies show, for example, that oleuropein and hydroxytyrosol can help protect against heart disease, cancer, and brain degeneration. [1, 2, 3]

One of the most exciting things about Sirtfoods is that sirtuins cause fat to be burned and muscle mass to increase, which is why they are sometimes known as 'skinny' genes. This means that by eating more Sirtfoods, we can become leaner and fitter without having to diet or take extra exercise.

Other top Sirtfoods are chili, capers, celery, kale, red onions, red wine, rocket, and walnuts. A large salad with olives, chili, rocket, and a dressing made with extra-virgin olive oil is a great way to have a Sirtfood meal; or try drizzling olive oil over steamed kale and adding a sprinkle of chili and a squeeze of lemon. And now that the festive season is on the horizon, I for one will be enjoying a glass of red wine with a bowl of spicy olives before dinner.

8. DARK CHOCOLATE (85% COCOA)

Dark Chocolate along with Red Wine has captured the most attention amongst the top-20 Sirtfoods. In fact, it is really Cocoa that is rich in a specific group of polyphenols called flavanols, especially epicatechin that is the actual Sirtfood.

In clinical studies, flavanol-rich cocoa has shown impressive health benefits spanning many of the major afflictions of modern times. This is especially so in relation to heart health, where cocoa has shown promise in lowering blood pressure, improving blood flow to the heart, preventing blood clots, and reducing inflammation. Benefits may also extend to aiding in the prevention of diseases such as diabetes and cancer and enhancing memory performance.

So what chocolate exactly are we talking about here? Alas, the bulk of confectionary chocolate won't deliver these profound benefits. Those products tend to be more sugar and milk than anything else. As a consequence, the prevailing wisdom dictates that the darker the chocolate, the high the level of beneficial cocoa flavanols will be.

To be counted as a Sirtfood we are talking about chocolate with 85 percent cocoa solids. But in reality, that is a gross over-simplification. Much of the dark chocolate that we turn to as a 'healthy treat' has undergone a form of processing known as alkalizing (or 'dutching'), which greatly diminishes the flavanol content, and thus the health benefits.

While in the USA these products are clearly labeled 'processed with alkali', unfortunately in the UK and in many other countries no such labeling requirements exist. This makes it difficult to know which brand to choose to reap the true benefits of the Sirtfood cocoa.

9. MATCHA GREEN TEA

Matcha is a type of tea that's far less processed than regular green tea because the leaves are never heated and kept under shade to preserve the natural nutrients found in the leaves. Regular green tea goes through much more processing during production and is also left to dry in the sun, versus in the shade like matcha is. Matcha green tea is a bright, green powder that's also stirred into warmed liquid instead of boiling and brewing methods used when making regular green tea. Since you're consuming the leaves whole in a milder powder with matcha, you're also taking in more nutrients than just throwing the leaves away in a tea bag or straining them out in a strainer as you would with regular tea.

How Does Matcha Taste?

Like all green tea, matcha has slightly grass notes, but with a much richer, almost buttery flavor. It's especially tasty when blended with some non-dairy milk and stevia, along with a little vanilla extract.

Superfood Benefits of Matcha:

Matcha green tea far outranks even some of the most powerful superfoods we know of today. It contains over six times the antioxidants in goji berries, seven times the antioxidants in dark chocolate, 17 times more antioxidants than blueberries, and 60 times the antioxidants found in spinach. And that's just in one teaspoon!

Matcha contains 137 times more of the popular antioxidant EGCG found in regular green tea. EGCG is a part of the antioxidant family known as catechins, which have been linked to better heart health, a healthy metabolism, and improved aging.

Matcha is a great tool to improve your workouts since it's energizing and anti-inflammatory.

The beautiful bright green tea has even been found to prevent cancer because the antioxidants in the tea are so high, they help fight off immune system invaders known as free radicals.

Matcha is five times higher in chlorophyll than regular tea. Chlorophyll is the green pigment found in plants that can help give you clear skin, protect your blood and heart, and also help prevent joint inflammation.

One glass of matcha green tea is equal to the amount of nutrition found in 10 cups of regular green tea.

Matcha green tea has been found to raise the metabolism, provides a long stream of energy versus a crash you get with coffee, and possibly help with weight management. Of course, matcha isn't a replacement for an unhealthy diet, but it is a much smarter, holistic way to raise your metabolism and gain energy.

Matcha also lowers anxiety due to the high, raw amounts of L-theanine found in matcha. L-theanine is an amino acid that promotes a state of relaxation and is the reason regular green tea is thought of as a calming beverage.

Matcha only contains 35 milligrams of caffeine per teaspoon, which is almost a third less than a cup of regular black coffee.

Sounds pretty amazing for a tea, right? That's because matcha, like all plant-based foods, has unique properties that make it special in its own light. Remember that matcha isn't a quick-fix magic pill to perfect health, but it sure beats out other teas and is a better, less-processed option.

Enjoy Matcha Green Tea:

Traditional use: Matcha can be enjoyed the same way you would use regular green tea, you just have to brew it a bit differently. Boil a cup and a half of water, pour it in your favorite tea mug, and let it sit for 3-5 minutes.

Then whisk in 1/2 teaspoon of matcha green tea powder. You'll notice it starts to foam a bit, and this is completely natural. You can also add a little non-dairy milk if you like, which will give it a creamier flavor. Or blend it all together in your blender to make it frothier like cafe-style beverages.

Other uses: Matcha is also amazing in a green smoothie. You can use it to replace your normal green superfood powder with a pinch, or just use it in any other regular smoothie. Since it's so high in nutrition, you don't need a lot of it to get the health benefits. A half to a whole teaspoon is plenty.

You can also use matcha in energy bites, vegan ice cream, truffles, and even bake brownies and cupcakes. Or, keep things simple and blend it with some ice and non-dairy milk to make an iced matcha latte. Get creative and see how you can incorporate matcha into your life!

Where to Find Matcha and What to Look For:

It's important not to buy just any old brand of matcha tea. Many brands market matcha tea that isn't true matcha. The better brands will be slightly pricier than cheap versions you find at the grocery store, and this indicates their higher quality. Check the label on all matcha you buy. It should only include 100 % matcha green tea leaves and preferably be organic and ceremonial grade, which indicates it's produced in the same, minimally-processing method of green tea consumed in Japan and will ensure it contains no pesticides.

The color should also be a bright green, not a muddy greenish-brown color, which indicates it's been more heavily processed or is a cheaper variety of matcha.

Most matcha is sold in 2-4 ounce containers and ranges anywhere from $15.00-$50.00 per container. These are definitely not cheap but will last at least three months if you use a half teaspoon per day.

10. BUCKWHEAT

Despite its recent rise to prominence, buckwheat is actually an ancient grain with a long history. It has been eaten in Asian and Eastern European countries for centuries, but is now becoming increasingly popular in the west due to its many health benefits.

While buckwheat is often thought of as a cereal grain, it is actually a fruit seed that is related to rhubarb and sorrel. However, because its seeds are rich in complex carbohydrates, it is sometimes referred to as a pseudo-cereal.

While it is not a true grain, it can be used like one in cooking and is a delicious alternative to couscous, bulgur wheat, rice and pasta.

Buckwheat is super healthy, very versatile and, despite its name, it's not actually related to wheat. It is naturally gluten free and should, therefore, be safe to eat for those with coeliac disease and gluten sensitivities.

Buckwheat also comes in several different forms: buckwheat seeds (often called buckwheat groats, or just buckwheat), noodles, pasta and flour. The groats are available completely raw or sprouted and are also available toasted. The toasted buckwheat groats are commonly referred to as kasha and have an earthier, nuttier flavor than the raw buckwheat.

Why is buckwheat so healthy?

Buckwheat is high in protein and fiber. It is rich in many trace minerals, including manganese, magnesium, and copper, and is a good source of the B vitamins. It also contains relatively few calories (66 calories for an 80g cooked portion, 40g uncooked) and practically no fat. Buckwheat also ranks low on the glycaemic scale. In fact, buckwheat is so packed with nutrients and antioxidants that it is often referred to as a "superfood".

Diets that contain buckwheat have been linked to a lowered risk of developing high cholesterol and high blood pressure and buckwheat may even help weight loss, reduce food cravings, and improve diabetes.

It is an excellent source of plant-based protein, meaning buckwheat is a great choice for vegetarian and vegan diets.

How do you cook buckwheat?

Buckwheat is actually incredibly easy to cook, but our biggest piece of advice would be: be wary of following the packet instructions! The instructions on my packet of Tesco Buckwheat advised me to cook it for 30 minutes – well after 20 minutes it was a horrible tasting mush. Goodness knows what would have happened after 30 minutes! Less is obviously better. Our advice is to cook the buckwheat for 10 to 15 minutes in plenty of boiling water and drain. That's it.

Whether you cook it for 10 or 15 minutes, it's a matter for personal taste – a bit like pasta. If you want to add a little extra taste to your buckwheat, try toasting it in the dry pan for 2 to 3 minutes first before adding the boiling water, this will give you some extra nutty flavors and a richer, deeper taste, but is not necessary if you are in a hurry. (Also, do be careful when adding the boiling water to the pan that's been toasting the buckwheat – it's liable to bubble up like a volcano!).

Buckwheat can be stored in the fridge for up to 3 days, making it a great one to cook up a big batch and use it for various salads throughout the week. It can also be frozen.

Does buckwheat taste nice?

Yes, but it can be a bit of an acquired taste. We would encourage you to persevere if you don't like it at first.

What do you do with buckwheat?

Buckwheat can be used in place of other carbs such as rice, couscous, potatoes, or pasta. It can be used as a side dish for a curry or stew. It can also be used instead of rice, bulgur wheat, or couscous in a salad.

Buckwheat can also be used instead of rice to make a risotto-style dish.

11. TURMERIC

This spice has been used since ancient times for its healing properties. Curcumin, its active ingredients, is a strong antioxidant and anti-inflammatory agent. This naturally occurring compound reduces inflammation in your body, which helps prevent arthritis, chronic pain, cancer, heart disease, and various degenerative conditions. Turmeric also enhances the body's antioxidant capacity, fights free radical damage, and improves brain function. This is one of the few foods containing BDNF (brain-derived neurotrophic factor), a protein that contributes to the growth, maturation, and survival of nerve cells.

12. WALNUTS

Eating too many nuts is often noted as one of the mistakes people make that stop them from losing weight. However, a new study suggests that walnuts may actually help you shed fat.

The study's lead scientist, Dr. Cheryl Rock of the University of California, San Diego School of Medicine compared various diets and was surprised to find, 'that even though walnuts are higher in fat and calories, the walnut-rich diet was associated with the same degree of weight loss as a lower fat diet.'

The research looked at 245 overweight women giving them one of three diets: A lower fat and higher carb diet, a lower carb and higher fat diet, and finally a walnut-rich, higher fat and lower carb diet.

Not only did the walnut-rich group see good weight loss, but they also saw a decrease in bad cholesterol and an increase in the good stuff!

Dr. Rock also explained: 'In addition to these findings, we hope to explore the effect of walnuts on satiety, as we believe satiety is a critical factor for maintaining weight loss.'

The Benefits Of Walnuts

Walnuts are naturally low in sugars, sodium, and packed with nutrients: healthy fats (plant omega-3 ALA), protein, fiber, antioxidants, as well as vitamins and minerals – folate, thiamin, magnesium, potassium, manganese, and copper.

Enjoying a handful of nuts (35g) as part of a healthy diet every day will contribute:

Protein – needed for growth and repair of tissues such as bones, muscles, and skin as well as being a plant protein source for vegetarians

Fiber – keeping you regular and helping control appetite

Plant omega 3s called Alpha Linoleic Acid (ALA) – just four or five walnuts a day can provide 100 percent of daily adult ALA needs

Antioxidants – which protect cells against free radical damage (polyphenols, copper, manganese)

Nutrients for energy production – thiamin, copper, manganese, magnesium

Nutrients for brain and neurological function – magnesium, copper, folate, thiamin

Folate – needed during pregnancy and for blood formation

Arginine an amino acid and polyphenol antioxidants – both help keep blood vessels elastic.

A healthy diet low in sodium, but with a variety of foods such as walnuts, can help reduce blood pressure and contribute to heart health.

13. ARUGULA (ROCKET)

Arugula is a lesser known cruciferous vegetable that provides many of the same benefits as other vegetables of the same family, which include broccoli, kale, and Brussels sprouts.

Arugula leaves, also known as rocket or roquette, are tender and bite-sized with a tangy flavor. Along with other leafy greens, arugula contains high levels of beneficial nitrates and polyphenols.

A 2014 review study found that high intakes of nitrate may lower blood pressure, reduce the amount of oxygen needed during exercise, and enhance athletic performance.

This article provides an in-depth look at the possible health benefits of arugula, a nutritional breakdown, how to add it to the diet, and possible health risks linked with eating arugula.

Benefits

Eating fruits and vegetables of all kinds reduces the risk of many adverse health conditions due to their high levels of antioxidants, fiber, and phytochemicals.

Research has specifically linked arugula and other cruciferous vegetables with the following health benefits:

1. Reduced cancer risk

While an overall healthful, vegetable-rich diet reduces a person's cancer risk, studies have shown that certain groups of vegetables can have specific anti-cancer benefits.

A 2017 meta-analysis linked eating more cruciferous vegetables with reduced total cancer risk, along with a reduction in all-cause mortality.

Cruciferous vegetables are a source of glucosinolates, which are sulfur-containing substances. Glucosinolates may be responsible for the plants' bitter taste and their cancer-fighting power. The body breaks down glucosinolates into a range of beneficial compounds, including sulforaphane.

Researchers have found that sulforaphane can inhibit the enzyme histone deacetylase (HDAC), which is involved in the progression of cancer cells. The ability to stop HDAC enzymes could make foods that contain sulforaphane a potentially significant part of cancer treatment in the future.

Reports have linked diets high in cruciferous vegetables with a reduced risk of breast cancer, colorectal cancer, lung cancer, prostate cancer, and more. However, the research is limited, and scientists need more high-quality evidence before confirming these benefits.

Easily recognized cruciferous vegetables include broccoli, cauliflower, kale, cabbage, Brussels sprouts, and turnips. Less well known types include arugula, bok choy, and watercress.

2. Osteoporosis prevention

Arugula is high in several key nutrients for bone health, including calcium and vitamin K.

The Office of Dietary Statistics states that vitamin K is involved in bone metabolism and that a deficiency can increase the risk of bone fracture. Leafy green vegetables are one of the primary dietary sources of vitamin K.

One cup of arugula provides 21.8 micrograms (mcg) of vitamin K, which goes towards the adult Food and Drug Administration's (FDA) daily value (DV) recommendation of 80 mcg for adults.

Adequate vitamin K consumption improves bone health by playing an essential role in bone mineralization and helps to improve how the body absorbs and excretes calcium, which is another crucial nutrient for bone health.

Arugula also contributes to a person's daily need for calcium, providing 32 milligrams (mg) per cup, going towards the DV of 1,000 mg for adults.

3. Diabetes

Several review studies have found that eating vegetables reduces a person's risk of developing type 2 diabetes. A review study from 2016 reports that leafy green vegetables are especially beneficial.

One test tube study showed that arugula extract had antidiabetic effects in mouse skeletal muscle cells. They produced this effect by stimulating glucose uptake in the cells.

Plus, arugula and other cruciferous vegetables are a good source of fiber, which helps to regulate blood glucose and may reduce insulin resistance. High fiber foods make people feel fuller for longer, meaning they can help tackle overeating.

4. Heart health

Vegetable intake, specifically cruciferous vegetables, has protective effects on the heart.

A 2017 meta-analysis reports that diets rich in cruciferous vegetables, salads, and green leafy vegetables have links with a reduced risk of cardiovascular disease.

In addition, a 2018 study published in the Journal of the American Heart Association reported that consuming a diet high in cruciferous vegetables could reduce atherosclerosis in older women. Atherosclerosis is a common condition where plaque builds up in the arteries, increasing a person's risk of cardiovascular problems.

The heart protective effects of these vegetables may be due to their high concentration of beneficial plant compounds, including polyphenols and organosulfur compounds.

14. BIRD'S EYE CHILI

The Sirtfood Bird's-Eye Chillies contain the major sirtuin-activating nutrients Luteolin and Myricetin.

Bird's-eye chilies (sometimes referred to as 'Thai chilies') are one of the top 20 Sirtfoods and appear regularly in the recipe sections(here and here) of this website. If you are not used to spicy food, it is suggested you start with half the chili amount stated in the recipe, as well as deseeding your chili before use. You can adjust the heat to your preference throughout the diet.

The chili originated in the Americas and has been part of the human diet since at least 7500 BC. Explorer Christopher Columbus brought it back to Spain in the 15th century and its cultivation spread rapidly through the rest of the world. Its pungent heat is designed as a plant defense mechanism to cause discomfort and dissuade predators from feasting on it, yet many relish adding it to their eating patterns.

There are more than 200 varieties, colored anything from yellow to green to red to black, and varying in heat from mildly warm to mouth-blisteringly hot.

Bird's- Eye Chillies boasts much greater sirtuin-activating credentials than the milder standard chilies that are more commonly used.

Bird's-Eye chilies are known for weight reducing qualities. They can play a key role in increasing the metabolism of the body by increasing your body temperature. Faster metabolism, proper digestion, and waste expulsion can decrease the chance of fat accumulation in the body.

The chemical compound present in Bird's-Eye chili which results in the burning sensation is called Capsaicin. The effects of this compound can vary among individuals. However, most common is a burning sensation of the mouth, throat, and stomach upon ingestion.

It's not just the heat of chilies but the way they enhance the flavors of other ingredients.

15. LOVAGE

Lovage, a member of the parsley family, is a widely-used herb in parts of Europe and southwest Asia. It's an extremely versatile plant possessing flavors of both celery and parsley but much stronger. Lovage is delicious and also extremely high in the sirtuin-activating compound quercetin and is one of the main ingredients of the Sirtfood Green Juice. Lovage offers a number of health benefits, including supporting kidney health, fighting harmful organisms, and supporting joint health.

Here are some of the well-researched benefits of Lovage.

1. Lovage Fights the Risk of Kidney Stones

Lovage is an aquaretic or a type of diuretic that encourages urination without electrolyte loss. The increased urination flushes the urinary tract to potentially help avoid kidney stones.

2. Lung Support

Traditional herbal medicine uses lovage to loosen phlegm in the lungs, which in turn improves airflow, breathing, and oxygen intake. In one trial eucalyptol, the active chemical compound in lovage that reduces lung irritation, produced significant, positive results within four days

3. Soothes Rough Spots

It turns out lovage is loaded with compounds that may soothe rough patches in the body. Compounds in lovage that provide this benefit include limonene, eugenol, and quercetin. Studies involving limonene have shown it provides soothing effects throughout the body, although it has been especially noted to help reduce issues associated with colitis.

4. Promotes Healthy Skin

Lovage is recommended as a natural way to fight skin conditions like dermatitis and acne. The exact mechanism of action is not fully understood, but traditional skincare approaches include lovage in their routines.

5. Fights Harmful Organisms

Scientists have found lovage to be one of the most potent extracts against organisms like E. coli, Salmonella, H. pylori, and H. influenza.

6. Eases Digestion and Relieves Gas

The soothing benefits of lovage are very effective and it's even a great remedy to soothe the digestive tract, reduce bloating, and relieve gas.

7. Supports Joint Health

The herb is considered a natural remedy for joint discomfort associated with gout and rheumatic swelling of the joints. In addition, it doesn't cause any terrible side effects.

8. Natural Allergy Support

The soothing effects of lovage naturally help fight the symptoms of allergies. But when it comes to allergies, lovage goes a bit farther. Quercetin, a compound present in lovage, inhibits histamine release and alleviates skin irritation typically caused by sensitivity to environmental irritants.

9. Menstrual Support

Among its many traditional uses, lovage is reported to provide relief from menstrual discomfort. Its high nutrient density combined with its powerful soothing benefits may explain why adding lovage to the diet prior to the beginning of a menstrual cycle may support well-being.

10. Excellent for Recipes

Lovage is a wonderful addition to your favorite recipes, adding taste, and increasing your meal's nutrient value. It's often used as a replacement for celery, although it's more pungent so most recipes recommend using about half the amount of the celery called for. The leaves make an excellent salad, and the seeds are used as a spice and often sprinkled over salads and soups. Lovage can even be brewed as an herbal tea. It's rich in B-complex vitamins, essential for energy, and vitamin C which supports skin and immune system health.

Lovage is safe, natural and can easily be found as a portion of food or herbal supplement!

16. MEDJOOL DATES

MEDJOOL DATES are a type of tree fruit that originates in the Middle East and North Africa, but they can be cultivated with some success in a number of desert-like regions around the world. Dates, in general, make up an important part of Middle Eastern cuisine, but Medjools particularly are prized for their large size, their sweet taste, and their juicy flesh even when dried. They are often enjoyed on their own as a snack or as a flavoring element within a larger meal or baked confection.

The difference from Other Sorts of Dates

There are many different varieties of dates, though all share some basic characteristics. They grow on date palm trees, for instance, and are native to hot, arid climates. Their fruit can be eaten fresh but is more commonly dried, which lengthens its lifespan and prevents early spoilage. Medjool dates are widely regarded as the "best" variety of dates. They are certainly the largest and are usually also the most expensive to buy. Many consumers believe that they have the richest flavor as well.

Medjools are often informally known as the "king of dates," the "diamond of dates," or the "crown jewel of dates" in reference to their elevated position. They are what is known as a "soft" date. The fruits are usually categorized as soft, dry, or semi-dry in reference to their texture and taste. Soft dates are usually considered to be the most exquisite in part because of how much harder they are to grow, as well as how much more susceptible they are to lose by birds and insects.

Taste Basics Of Medjool Dates

Most people describe Medjool dates as having a rich, almost caramel-like taste, and mentions of honey and cinnamon are also common. They are usually served dried, but this drying happens naturally in most cases. The most traditional way to prepare dates of any kind is to allow them to ripen and then sun dry while still connected to the tree. When picked at the right time, medjools need no additional treatment or care before serving.

Nutritional Profile

Medjool dates only contain about 66 calories each. They are a good source of fiber and contain high levels of the essential minerals, potassium, magnesium, copper, and manganese. Most do contain a significant amount of fruit sugar, but this can make them a good alternative to more caloric desserts. In the Middle East where they grow wild, they are a popular food for nomadic travelers as they provide a lot of energy and healthful nutrients with the added benefit of being readily available.

How to Enjoy Medjool Dates

One of the easiest ways to enjoy Medjool dates is to eat them on their own, either as an independent snack or alongside other finger foods like hard cheeses, crackers, and crusty pieces of bread. The dates do contain a pit, but it is big and generally very easy to remove.

The fruit's large size also lends well to stuffing once the pit has been removed. Walnuts, almonds, and honeycomb are some of the more traditional things that cooks can put inside, but there is a lot of room for creativity. Some people put other fruits, small pieces of chocolate, or savory meats into the pit cavity in order to create a one-of-a-kind taste.

Use in Cooking

Medjool dates also feature in a number of recipes. Many North African stews call for sliced Medjools, for instance, and they are commonly mixed with yoghurt for breakfast in countries like Iraq and Iran. They add sweetness to a number of cooked meat dishes and can also be incorporated into the batter of many different loaves of bread and baked goods.

Where They Grow

Date palms that give rise to Medjool fruit are believed to be indigenous to the North African coast and Arabic Peninsula. Fossil evidence suggests that the fruits were enjoyed by ancient people in countries as far apart as Saudi Arabia and Morocco, and the land between these countries remains the primary growing area. Many California farmers have had some luck cultivating the trees, however, as have some people in Australia. They are often much harder to grow than other date varieties because of how sensitive the fruits are to air quality and soil moisture. They often take a tremendous amount of work to grow on demand, which is part of the reason for their relatively high price.

Cultivation at Home

The most basic way to grow a Medjool date palm is to plant a pit and wait for it to sprout, though this is also the most time-consuming and potentially frustrating method. It can take up to 20 years for a sprouted pit to yield a tree that actually bears fruit. Home gardeners wanting to try their hand at growing Medjools are usually better served by purchasing established plants from nurseries or local distributors or grafting branches from existing palms onto new plants. Trees typically need a lot of care, as well as close attention to sunlight and soil quality, in order to thrive. Some gardeners have had success cultivating the plants in indoor greenhouses, though the best fruits tend to come from trees exposed to more natural outdoor settings.

17. RED CHICORY

The red chicory is a top 20 Sirtfood. As with the Sirtfood onion, red is best but the yellow variety of chicory is also a Sirtfood.

The red variety can be harder to find but yellow is a perfectly suitable alternative. If you are wondering how to add chicory to your diet, you can add its leaves to a salad where the tart flavor adds crunch to an extra virgin olive oil-based dressing.

Chicory does belong to the Asteraceae family with sunflowers and dandelions and has been used throughout Europe for millennia as both a food and a medicine. Although chicory contains no huge amounts of any one nutrient, it can claim small amounts of the whole spectrum of vitamins and minerals, the most prominent being vitamins C and A, selenium, manganese, fiber, potassium, and phosphorus, as well as the sirtuin-activating nutrient Luteolin.

Chicory can be eaten raw or cooked. Although called chicory in the UK, it is more commonly known as Chicon or Witloof (meaning white leaf) in Belgium and is called Endive in the US.

Chicory is a woody, herbaceous plant that has a wealth of researched health benefits. They include the ability to ease digestive problems, prevent heartburn, reduce arthritic pains, detoxify the liver and gallbladder, prevent bacterial infections, boost the immune system, and reduce the chance of heart disease. It is also a natural sedative and can protect against kidney stones, and benefit attempts to lose weight. All in all, this small plant is a powerful addition to any diet.

Chicory is probably better known to many people for its roots which can be roasted, ground, and used as a coffee substitute. Chicory is native to France, where it has long been loved for culinary reasons so it's only natural that's where it originated.

18. BLUEBERRIES

Blueberries are an excellent source of vitamin C, vitamin K, manganese, copper, and dietary fiber. They also have the highest antioxidant content of all berries. These popular Sirtfoods boost immunity and neutralize the free radicals that can damage cellular structures. Low in calories and carbs, they're ideal for dieters. Recent studies suggest that blueberries may help reduce stomach fat and risk factors for metabolic syndrome. Rich in calcium, they also strengthen your bones and prevent osteoporosis.

19. ZCAPERS

Capers boast powerful anti-inflammatory effects, offering a cocktail of vitamins, minerals, and antioxidants. They have only 23 calories per 100 grams and provide large amounts of calcium, potassium, vitamin K, riboflavin, iron, copper, and phytonutrients. Quercetin and rutin, the key antioxidants in capers, have strong analgesic, antibacterial, and anti-carcinogenic properties. Rutin helps prevent and treat hemorrhoids, improves circulation, and reduces bad cholesterol levels in obese patients. Quercetin inhibits tumor growth and boosts immune function. The best way to use capers is by adding them to salads, pasta, and casseroles.

20.COFFEE

The diet combines sirtfoods and calorie restriction, both of which may trigger the body to produce higher levels of sirtuins.

The Sirtfood Diet book includes meal plans and recipes to follow, but there are plenty of other Sirtfood Diet recipe books available.

The diet's creators claim that following the Sirtfood Diet will lead to rapid weight loss, all while maintaining muscle mass and protecting you from chronic disease. Once you have completed the diet, you are encouraged to continue including sirtfoods and the diet's signature green juice into your regular diet.

These aforementioned are the 20 sirtfood diet. The diet is divided into two phases; the initial phase lasts one week and involves restricting calories to 1000kcal for three days, consuming three sirtfood green juices, and one meal rich in sirtfoods each day. The juices include kale, celery, rocket, parsley, green tea, and lemon. Meals include turkey escalope with sage, capers and parsley, chicken and kale curry and prawn stir-fry with buckwheat noodles. From days four to seven, energy intakes are increased to 1500kcal comprising of two sirtfood green juices and two sirtfood-rich meals a day.

Although the diet promotes healthy foods, it's restrictive in both your food choices and daily calories, especially during the initial stages. It also involves drinking juice, with the amounts suggested during phase one exceeding the current daily guidelines.

The second phase is known as the maintenance phase which lasts 14 days where steady weight loss occurs. The authors believe it's a sustainable and realistic way to lose weight. However, focusing on weight loss is not what the diet is all about – it's designed to be about eating the best foods nature has to offer. Long term they recommend eating three balanced sirtfood rich meals a day along with one sirtfood green juice.

Dietitian Emer Delaney says:

'At first glance, this is not a diet I would advise for my clients. Aiming to have 1000kcal for three consecutive days is extremely difficult and I believe the majority of people would be unable to achieve it. Looking at the list of foods, you can see they are the sort of items that often appear on a 'healthy food list', however it would be better to encourage these as part of a healthy balanced diet. Having a glass of red wine or a small amount of chocolate occasionally won't do us any harm - I wouldn't recommend them on a daily basis. We should also be eating a mixture of different fruits and vegetables and not just those on the list.

'In terms of weight loss and boosting metabolism, people may have experienced a seven pound weight loss on the scales, but in my experience, this will be fluid. Burning and losing fat takes time so it is extremely unlikely this weight loss is a loss of fat. I would be very cautious of any diet that recommends fast and sudden weight loss as this simply isn't achievable and will more than likely be a loss of fluid. As soon as people return to their regular eating habits, they will regain the weight. Slow and steady weight loss is the key and for this, we need to restrict calories and increase our activity levels. Eating balanced regular meals made up of low GI foods, lean protein, fruit and vegetables, and keeping well hydrated is the safest way to lose weight.'

MATCHA GREEN TEA OR COFFEE

There have been recent media stories downgrading the health benefits of coffee. Meanwhile, health experts and celebrities are touting the benefits of matcha green tea as one of the world's best beverages for your taste buds and your body. Whilst both coffee and green tea are both Sirtfoods there is a piece of growing evidence and publicity around the benefits of matcha green tea.

1. Matcha's Antioxidants vs. Coffee's Acidity

Matcha green tea is loaded with antioxidants that are known to fight oxidative stress, and this tea is one of the few foods known to possess a special type of antioxidant: catechins. A Harvard research study concluded that green tea was the best food source of catechins, and matcha green tea ranked the highest of all in a University of Colorado Springs' comparison study between matcha and common green tea. Specifically, matcha was 137 times higher in catechins!

On the other hand, coffee has a very acidic reputation. This acidity can exacerbate heartburn and acid reflux. Contrary to popular belief, decaffeinated coffee can prove to be more acidic than regular coffee. One wonders if America's love for coffee and overuse of antacids are related.

2. Matcha Lowers Cancer Risk vs. Coffee's Acrylamide Carcinogens

Research shows that the consumption of matcha green tea may lower your risk for multiple types of cancer. In a study conducted on green tea and colon and rectal cancer, 69,710 Chinese women had a 57% lower risk of colorectal cancer. Another study showed that when Japanese men drank 5 or more cups of green tea per day they lowered their risk of prostate cancer by 48%!

The State of California keeps a list of chemicals that could cause cancer. Among them is listed acrylamide, a carcinogen linked to coffee. This chemical is produced when the coffee beans are roasted. California caused uproar recently when they began to require coffee retailers and businesses to warn customers that coffee contained acrylamide with potential carcinogens. Research does not show an association between cancer and the dietary consumption of coffee thus far, but the mere mention of the word carcinogen should be a cause for concern especially in a culture that consumes coffee on a massive scale.

3. Matcha Promotes Weight Loss vs. Coffee May Increase Belly Fat

In a study published in the American Journal of Clinical Nutrition, researchers wanted to analyze the effects of green tea upon weight loss. One group of participants was given 690 milligrams of green tea and another group was given only 22 milligrams. At the conclusion of 12 weeks, the first group of participants' body fat was significantly lower than the other group after taking BMI and a variety of other factors into consideration. The researchers concluded that catechins are great at burning fat.

Unfortunately for coffee lovers, the caffeine in coffee increases stress hormones in the body such as cortisol and adrenaline. Cortisol has been linked to an increase of visceral fat or what is also known as belly fat.

4. Matcha Boosts Immune Function vs. Coffee Decreases Immune Function

The high antioxidant content found in matcha green tea directly boosts your immune system. The EGCG found in matcha helps your body to produce more T-cells to fight infection. Matcha is also naturally anti-bacterial, anti-inflammatory, and detoxifying.

Caffeine can increase your stress hormones, but did you know that increased stress hormones result in suppressed immune function? Your body will get a kick from that coffee at first, but if you abuse caffeine it will deliver a swift kick to your pants when you're not looking.

5. Matcha Calms Your Anxiety vs. Coffee Can Increase It

Matcha contains the amino acid, l-theanine, which promotes a sense of calm. Research has shown l-theanine to be beneficial to patients diagnosed with anxiety because it increases levels of dopamine and GABA in the brain.

In contrast, coffee actually interferes with GABA metabolism. This transmitter is crucial in the regulation of mood and stress management. Caffeine prevents GABA from binding to GABA receptor sites.

Keep in mind that matcha's health benefits can be negated by the addition of sugar. If you are looking for a quality matcha green tea mix you can make at home, we highly recommend the Jade Leaf Matcha Green Tea Powder.

Coffee Boosts Weight Loss?

Coffee as one of the top 20 Sirtfoods continues to receive attention with new research into its health benefits.

Coffee will boost your weight loss, according to a new diet book that reveals how to harness the joys of coffee to shed pounds. Dr. Bob Arnot, author of The Coffee Lover's Diet: Change Your Coffee, Change Your Life, claims that the simple act of drinking a cup of coffee can improve your overall health as well as whittle your waistline. His recommendations about coffee are backed up by recent studies showing the benefits of drinking that morning cup of coffee.

Dr. Arnot described a cup of coffee as "the easiest way to change your health." And for those who want to focus on weight loss, the physician emphasized the benefits.

"When you drink a cup of hot coffee, you are burning another hundred calories a day and that's significant."

As for how coffee helps the body to burn fat faster, it stimulates the nervous system. In turn, that system signals the fat cells to break down fat. Beyond helping the body to burn fat, coffee can lower the perception of muscle pain from exercise.

Adding exercise to the weight loss equation can help, according to Dr. Arnot. He recommends sipping coffee one hour before working out as a way to improve your exercise regimen.

The coffee gives you the motivation to exercise. It also gives you the fuel and the power," explained the diet expert. "It feels easier to exercise, you can go longer, harder and you are going to be taking that weight off."

How much coffee should you drink daily for the maximum rewards? Dr. Arnot suggests sipping four to six cups of coffee a day.

Beyond weight loss, the physician noted that coffee has been shown to help reduce the risk of cancer and diabetes as well as prevent heart disease and even depression. The driving force behind depression and heart disease and so many diseases is inflammation, and coffee is a powerful ultimate anti-inflammatory drink.

Black Coffee in the Morning and Green Tea in the Afternoon

As well as the recommended daily servings of green juices, you can consume other fluids freely throughout all phases of the Sirtfood diet. These should include non-caloric drinks, preferably plain water, black coffee, and green tea. Both coffee and green tea are Sirtfoods and there is now considerable research now that drinking both are linked with numerous health benefits.

We recommend that coffee be drunk black, without adding milk as some researchers have found that the milk can reduce the absorption of the beneficial sirtuin-activating nutrients. The same has been found for green tea although adding some lemon juice actually increases the assimilation of the sirtuin-activators.

Mounting research suggests coffee may offer protection against a number of health concerns, including cancer, type 2 diabetes, heart disease, and Parkinson's. It also has athletic performance-enhancing benefits

Green tea has also been shown to improve heart, bone, and vision health, and may protect against type 2 diabetes and cancer. Long-term consumption may also promote weight loss

Quality is paramount for both coffee and tea. The healthiest coffee is an organic dark roast, ground from fresh whole coffee beans, consumed "black." Also, look for organic tea grown in a pristine environment.

While the research suggests you can have upwards of five cups of coffee per day without adverse effects, we believe this may be too much for many, especially with adrenal fatigue being so common. One way to balance the risks and benefits would be to limit your coffee consumption to one or two cups in the morning and drinking green tea in the afternoon. Also, remember that to achieve therapeutic benefits from coffee, it needs to be:

Organic: Most coffee produced today is heavily contaminated with pesticides. It's actually one of the most heavily sprayed crops grown. So, any coffee you consume should be organic, pesticide-free coffee.

Fresh whole bean: You'll want to purchase coffee in whole bean form and then grind it yourself to prevent rancidity. Pre-ground coffee may be rancid by the time you drink it.

Properly dried and roasted: The coffee should smell and taste fresh, not stale. If your coffee does not have a pleasant aroma, it is likely rancid and poor quality. Darker roasts may provide greater health benefits and be easier on your stomach than light roasts.

Black: Drink your coffee black, without sugar or cream. Add sugar and you'll certainly ruin any of the benefits discussed above by spiking your insulin levels and causing insulin resistance.

Tea also has its issues. Green tea plants are known to be especially effective at absorbing lead from the soil, which is then taken up into the plants' leaves.

Areas with excessive industrial pollution, such as China (where nearly 90 percent of the world's green tea is produced), may contain substantial amounts of lead.

While the lead in the tea leaves is not thought to leach very effectively into the tea, if you're consuming Matcha green tea (which contains the entire ground tea leaf), it's especially important that it comes from Japan instead of China.

Both black and green teas are also naturally high in fluoride, even if organically grown without pesticides. This is because the plant readily absorbs fluoride thorough its root system, including naturally occurring fluoride in the soil.

So, as with coffee, when selecting tea, opt for organic (to avoid pesticides), grown in a pristine environment (to avoid fluoride, heavy metals, and other toxins from contaminated soil and water). A clean growing environment is essential to producing a pure, high-quality tea.

MEAT IN SIRTFOOD DIET

Sirtfood was a breakthrough food regime a few years ago, and was the darling diet with the broadsheet press at the time. If you missed it, the headlines are that it includes red wine, chocolate and coffee. Far less publicised and attention grabbing, (but equally good news in our opinion) is the fact that the answer to the question, 'can you eat meat on the sirt food diet?', is a resounding, yes. The diet plan not only includes a good healthy portion of meat, it goes on to suggest that protein is an essential inclusion in a Sirtfood-based diet to reap maximum benefit. We're not advocating this as some meat heavy diet (we still remember the bad breath from Atkins), it's actually very vegetarian friendly and caters for pretty much everyone, which is what makes it so sensible an option to us.

Eating Meat on the Sirtfood Diet

So what is the Sirtfood diet? It was developed by nutritionists Aidan Goggins and Glen Matten, following a pilot study at the exclusive KX Gym, (Daniel Craig, Madonna and a whole host of other celebs are allegedly members) where they are both consultants in Sloane Square, London. Participants in the trial lost 7lbs in the first seven days, in what the authors call the hyper-success stage. The science behind Sirtfoods falls out of a study in 2003 which found that a compound found in red wine, increased the lifespan of yeast. Ultimately, this led to the studies which explain the health benefits of red wine, and how (if drank moderately) people who drink red wine gain less weight.

Much of the science behind the Sirtfood diet is similar to that of 'fasting-diets' which have been popular for the past few years, whereby our bodies activate genes and our fat storage is switched off; our bodies essentially switch to survival mode, hence weight loss. The negatives to fasting-diets are the inevitable hunger that ensues, along with reduction in energy, irritable behaviour (when you're "hangry"), fatigue and muscle loss. The Sirtfood diet claims to counter those negatives, as it is not a fast, so hunger is not an issue, making it perfect for people who want to lead an active healthy lifestyle.

Sirtfoods are a (relatively newly discovered) group of foods that are powerful in activating the 'sirtuin' genes in our body, which are the genes activated in fasting diets. The book lists the top sirtfoods as birds-eye chill, buckwheat, capers, celery, coffee, green tea, and kale among others (buy the book if you want them all), and outlines a 21 day diet plan that is very high in the top 20 Sirtfoods. Crucially for us carnivores, the book goes on to suggest in the chapter entitled 'Sirtfoods for Life' that protein is essential to maintain metabolism and reduce loss of muscle when dieting. Leucine, is an amino acid found in protein, which compliments and actually enhances the actions of Sirtfoods. This means that the best way to eat Sirtfoods is by combining them with a chicken breast, steak or other source of leucine such as fish or eggs.

The book goes on to suggest that poultry can be eaten freely as much as you want (because it is an excellent source of protein, B vitamins, potassium and phosphorous), and that red meat (another excellent source of protein, iron, zinc and vitamin B12) can be eaten up to three times (750g raw weight) a week.

Overall we can totally see the benefit and appeal of the Sirtfood diet. Like pretty much any diet plan, it can be a faff getting all the ingredients, and and the 'Sirtfood green juice', which forms a core part of the first 14 days of the plan, is a pain to make and pretty expensive, but it does tastes surprisingly better than you'd expect. We only trialled a few days of the plan, and while there was noticeable weight loss, the real benefit of the book is the sensible approach of introducing Sirtfoods into your everyday meal planning.

PRINCIPLE OF THE SIRTFOOD DIET

The Sirtfood diet is really not just another new trendy or fad diet. The principle of the diet is to bring about the knowledge of foods and how the health impact the nutrients you take in can be of benefit to your body. As Sirtfoods are natural they can be incorporated into your current diet – whether you favor a whole foods diet, paleo, or another diet – there's no disputing that these foods have remarkable health benefits.

Although the early stage of juicing and fasting seems just good for those who might want to lose a little weight quickly, the general aim of the Sirtfood diet is to include healthier foods into your diet to increase your well being and boost your immune system.

So while the first seven days seem very difficult, the longer-term plan can work for everyone.

By focusing on introducing Sirtfood- rich ingredients into your everyday meals you can continue the fat burning whilst enjoying your regular favorites.

Sirtuins Activate Your Body's Wellness Genes

sirtuinsPeoples have always been fascinated by the 'Fountain of Youth' and how we can live longer and healthier lives. Well, the scientific community has an equal fascination with a family of genes called sirtuins. Each and every one of us houses sirtuins—often referred to as our skinny genes—and they are truly fascinating, holding the power to determine things like our ability to burn fat and stay slim, our susceptibility to disease, and even how long we are able to live.

So what makes sirtuins so powerful? Sirtuins are special because of their ability to switch our cells to a kind of survival mode—triggering a powerful recycling process that clears out cellular waste and burns fat. The benefits of this are pretty spectacular: Fat melts away and we become fitter, leaner, and healthier.

So how do we take advantage of sirtuins?

All this raises the question: What can we do to activate sirtuins and reap these amazing benefits? It is well-known that both fasting and exercise activate sirtuins. But alas, both demand an unwavering commitment to either food restriction or demanding exercise regimes. Cutting back on calories leaves us feeling fatigued, hungry, and decidedly cranky, and in the longer term can lead to muscle loss and a stagnant metabolism. As for exercise, the amount needed to be effective for weight loss requires a LOT of effort. Both can be hard to accomplish.

In 2013, the results of one of the most prestigious nutritional studies ever carried out were published. The premise of the study, called PREDIMED, was beautifully simple: It studied the difference between a Mediterranean-style diet supplemented with either extra-virgin olive oil or nuts and a more conventional modern diet. Results showed that after five years, heart disease and diabetes were slashed by an incredible 30 percent, along with major reductions in the risk of obesity in the Mediterranean diet group. This wasn't surprising, but when the study was investigated in greater detail it was discovered there was no difference in calorie, fat, or carbohydrate intake between the two groups. How do you explain that?

Not all (healthy) foods are created equal.

Research now shows that plants contain natural compounds called polyphenols that have immense benefits for our health. And when researchers analyzing PREDIMED investigated polyphenol consumption among the participants, the results were staggering. Over just the five-year period, those who consumed the highest levels of polyphenols had 37 percent fewer deaths compared to those who ate the least.

But not all polyphenols are equal. Data out of Harvard University from over 124,000 individuals showed that only certain polyphenols were helpful for weight control. Similarly, a study of almost 3,000 twins found that a higher intake of only certain polyphenols was linked with less body fat and a healthier distribution of fat in the body. Polyphenols are undoubtedly a boon for staying slim and healthy, but if not all polyphenols are equal, then which are the best? Could it be those that research has shown to have the ability to switch on our sirtuin genes? The very same ones activated by fasting and exercise?

The pharmaceutical industry has been quick to exploit these sirtuin-activating nutrients, investing hundreds of millions to convert them into panacea drugs. For example, the popular diabetes drug metformin comes from a plant and activates our sirtuin genes. But until now they have been largely overlooked by the world of nutrition, to the detriment of our health and our waistlines.

What foods activate sirtuins?

With our interest piqued we put all the foods with the highest levels of sirtuin-activating polyphenols together into a special diet. This includes extra-virgin olive oil and walnuts, the specific inclusions in PREDIMED, as well as arugula, red onions, strawberries, red wine, dark chocolate, green tea, and coffee among many others. When we pilot tested it, the results were stunning. Participants lost weight, while either maintaining or even increasing their muscle mass. Best of all, people reported feeling great— brimming with energy, sleeping better, and with notable improvements in their skin.

And so the Sirtfood Diet was born, a revolutionary new way to activate sirtuins by eating delicious foods. A diet that doesn't involve calorie counting, cutting out carbs, or eating low fat. A diet of inclusion in which you reap the benefits from eating the foods your love. The Sirtfood Diet is challenging the status quo of healthy eating advice and what it really means to look and feel great. And all from eating our favorite foods!

Sirtfood Diet Green Juice

The Sirtfood Diet green juice is a major part of the Sirtfood Diet. It is included amongst the recipes included in the Best Sirtfood Recipes page so we thought it would be helpful to include the recipe separately here. Even if you have no intention of following the diet, the juice is packed full of nutrients and would be a great addition to a regular diet. One important thing to note: We have researched carefully and you absolutely need to make this in a juicer, NOT a blender (or a Nutribullet or food processor or anything else other than a juicer). We have tried both ways out and can report that the blended version is a nasty tasting sludge, the juiced version is a reasonably nice tasting juice!

The Sirtfood Diet green juice will keep for up to 3 days in the fridge, so it's well worth making up a big batch to save time. We usually make the juices up the night before to save time in the mornings. This Sirtfood Diet green juice is packed with nutrient rich Sirtfoods, great for anyone wanting a bit of a health boost and essential for anyone following the Sirtfood Diet.

INGREDIENTS

75g kale

30g rocket

5g parsley

2 celery sticks

½ green apple

1cm ginger

Juice of ½ lemon

½ teaspoon matcha green tea

METHOD

Juice all the ingredients apart from the lemon and the matcha green tea.

Squeeze the lemon juice into the green juice by hand.

Pour a small amount of green juice into a glass and stir in the matcha. Add the rest of the green juice into the glass and stir it again.

Drink straight away or save for later.

Sirtfood Diet And Exercise

With 52% of Americans confessing that they find it easier to do their taxes than to understand how to eat healthily, it's vital to introduce a form of eating that becomes a way of life rather than a one-off fad diet. For some of us it may not be that difficult to lose weight or retain a healthy weight, but the Sirtfood diet can help those who are struggling. But what about combining the Sirtfood diet with exercise, is it advisable to avoid exercise completely or introduce it once you have started the diet?

The SirtDiet Principles

With an estimated 650 million obese adults globally, it's important to find healthy eating and exercise regimes that are doable, don't deprive you of everything you enjoy, and don't require you to exercise all week. The Sirtfood diet does just that. The idea is that certain foods will active the 'skinny gene' pathways which are usually activated by fasting and exercise. The good news is that certain food and drink, including dark chocolate and red wine, contain chemicals called polyphenols that activate the genes that mimic the effects of exercise and fasting.

Exercise during the first few weeks

During the first week or two of the diet where your calorie intake is reduced, it would be sensible to stop or reduce exercise while your body adapts to fewer calories. Listen to your body and if you feel fatigued or have less energy than usual, don't work out. Instead ensure that you remain focused on the principles that apply to a healthy lifestyle such as including adequate daily levels of fibre, protein, and fruit and vegetables.

Once the diet becomes a way of life

When you do exercise it's important to consume protein ideally an hour after your workout. Protein repairs muscles after exercise reduces soreness and can aid recovery. There are a variety of recipes that include protein which will be perfect for post-exercise consumption, such as the sirt chili con carne or the turmeric chicken and kale salad. If you want something lighter you could try the sirt blueberry smoothie and add some protein powder for added benefit. The type of fitness you do will be down to you, but workouts at home will allow you to choose when to exercise, the types of exercises that suit you, and are short and convenient.

The Sirtfood diet is a great way to change your eating habits, lose weight, and feel healthier. The initial few weeks may challenge you but it's important to check which foods are best to eat and which delicious recipes suit you. Be kind to yourself in the first few weeks while your body adapts and takes exercise easily if you choose to do it at all. If you are already someone who does moderate or intense exercise then it may be that you can carry on as normal, or manage your fitness in accordance with the change in diet. As with any diet and exercise changes, it's all about the individual and how far you can push yourself.

Sirtfood Diet And The Science

Since time immemorial, humans have been fascinated by the pursuit of the mythical fountain of youth. Fast forward to the twenty-first century and sirtfood science nothing has changed, with enormous scientific interest now focused on a family of metabolism-regulating genes called sirtuin, and their potent actions that can fundamentally change how our cells function. These potent genes help us burn fat, become fitter and stave off disease, and ultimately could be the closest we ever get to turn back the clock.

But whether we like to think of them as 'skinny genes' or 'Peter Pan genes' as the media likes to coin them, what makes sirtuins special is their power to switch our cells into a survival mode. They do this by activating a powerful recycling process called autophagy, which clears out cellular waste and debris that builds up over time and is known to cause 'inflammaging'. The effects of this rejuvenation process are impressive: our cells return to a more youthful state where inflammation is quenched, fat burning increases and we once again feel like we did in our prime.

Which begs the million dollar question: how can we activate sirtuins and reap their remarkable benefits? There are two well-established methods: fasting and exercise. But as anyone will tell you, both can be grueling, and often not compatible with our busy and demanding twenty-first century lifestyle. Their downfalls are also well known. As many will attest, cutting back on calories makes us tired and 'hangry' (that formidably stressful combination of hungry and angry), and in the longer term can erode muscle and cause metabolism to stagnate. As for exercise, the amount needed to be effective for weight loss is verging on the herculean.

But what if there was a third, less grueling, way, a way that nature had always intended for us?

In 2013 the results of one of the biggest game changers in how we understand food was published. It was called PREDIMED, the largest, best-conducted nutrition study carried out in the modern era. Carried out on almost 7,500 people, PREDIMED asked a simple question: how did a Mediterranean-style diet supplemented with liberal extra virgin olive oil or nuts (especially walnuts) compare to a more conventional modern diet? The results were phenomenal. After 5 years, heart disease and diabetes were slashed by an astonishing 30%, accompanied by major reductions in inflammation as well as the risk of obesity. But what was most remarkable about this study was still to come. Upon further investigation, it transpired that there was no significant difference between the two groups in the number of calories, fat, or carbohydrates they consumed. These are all the usual measures we use when we determine how healthy a diet is. There was something altogether different going on, something that had yet to be considered by modern-day nutrition.

Plant foods – like extra virgin olive oil and walnuts – contain natural compounds called polyphenols, which research now shows have immense health benefits. When researchers analyzing PREDIMED investigated polyphenol consumption the results were staggering. Over just the five year period those who consumed the highest levels of polyphenols had 37% fewer deaths compared to those who consumed the least.

But not all polyphenols are equal. For instance, a study of almost 3,000 twins found that a higher intake of only certain polyphenols was linked with less body fat and healthier distribution of fat in the body. Specific polyphenols are undoubtedly a boon for staying slim and healthy, but which polyphenols are the best? Could it be those that research has shown to have the ability to switch on our sirtuin genes? The very same ones activated by fasting and exercise?

The pharmaceutical industry has been quick to jump on this idea, investing vast amounts of money to convert sirtuin activating nutrients into panacea drugs. Glaxo Smith Kline created a big stir when they paid almost a billion dollars for the rights to research the food nutrient resveratrol and develop it into a sirtuin activating drug. However, they fell victim to the pitfall of isolating a single nutrient and giving it at pharmaceutical doses, when research shows that the benefits come from a synergy of nutrients consumed at doses that it is possible to achieve through dietary sources.

Many will have heard of the most popular diabetes drug metformin, and many reading this will either take it or know someone who does. What you may not know is that it has natural plant origins, coming from the French lilac plant and was used as far back in the 1800s to treat diabetes. And whilst most popular drugs are associated with substantial side effects limiting their use, metformin has the accolade of being the first FDA approved drug to be investigated for extending life, so potent are its health benefits. And what causes such immense benefit? We now know it is because metformin does not act on blood sugar or macronutrients directly but works by activating the sirtuin gene pathway.

Paradoxically, whilst the pharmaceutical industry has been all over the phenomenal ability of plants to work at a genetic level to revolutionize health, it's an idea that has been almost entirely ignored in the nutrition world.

Researchers of the Sirtfood Diet set out to discover which foods contained the highest level of the specific polyphenols that had been shown in pharmaceutical screening studies to activate sirtuin genes. This culminated in the identification of the top 20 Sirtfoods, which we carefully put together into a special diet. This included extra virgin olive oil and walnuts, just like in PREDIMED, as well as arugula, red onions, strawberries, red wine, cocoa, chilies, turmeric, green tea, and coffee amongst other. When road tested this diet produced stunning results. Participants lost, on average, 7lbs in 7 days, whilst either maintaining or even increasing their muscle mass. Best of all people reported feeling great; brimming with energy, sleeping better and with notable improvements in their skin.

Whilst this represented a great kick start, it was the long-term results that truly showed the power of these plant foods as people lost in the range of 20 to 50 pounds over 12 weeks. This included many independent tests, including very recently a skeptical doctor testing it on national TV, with his patient losing a breath-taking 22 pounds in a mere four weeks.

But to focus only on weight loss is a disservice to our clinicians and the amazing foods that work at the very deepest genetic level of our cells to stop inflammation and aging. The Sirtfood Diet clinicians realized they had discovered something truly special with the life-changing health transformations, including people who reversed diabetes, heart disease, and auto-immune diseases and were able to give up their medicines. To date, hundreds of thousands of people around the world have now experienced the powerful effects of the Sirtfood Diet and the testimonials continue to flood in.

Without a doubt the benefits of a diet based around these foods show us that health is not defined by calorie counting, cutting out carbs, or banishing fat. Nature never intended us to be healthy based on what we cut out. Rather, nature intended for us to reap the benefits of a long and healthy life by indulging in its unrivaled food pharmacy.

A Great Juicer For The Sirtfood Diet

According to NBC News, fruit and vegetable juice can provide essential nutrients like vitamin C and potassium and can help prevent heart disease and even dementia. And while it's still important to eat whole fruits and vegetables to benefit from their roughage, juicing can be a great addition to your diet.

But with all the buzz about juicing, it can be hard to find a great juicer to help you add fresh fruit and vegetable juice to your regimen.

Juicers break down into two main categories: centrifugal and cold-press.

Centrifugal juicers shred and spin produce, resulting in a relatively speedy juicing experience. These models also tend to be a bit more affordable as well.

Cold-press juicers crush and twist produce against a screen to extract the juice. These tend to take slightly longer than their counterparts and also fall at a higher price point.

It's important to note that there are also manual juicers and citrus juicers on the market, but though the niche market for these models is small and they are often too specific or labor-intensive for a typical dieter.

Look for intuitive features and functions that help you stay on track

The biggest obstacle when it comes to incorporating fresh juice into your diet is keeping up with the regimen. Juicers can often be inefficient, hard to assemble or disassemble, or difficult to clean, making the juicing process something we'd rather avoid. The best juicer will facilitate your dietary needs with features and functions which will minimize these obstacles.

A variety of speed settings can ensure you're able to juice a variety of produce, from dry leafy greens to larger, watery foods.

Ease of assembly and disassembly is key to keeping you juicing on a daily basis. Before you use your machine, be sure it's not a nightmare to put together and take down!

A straightforward structure will also help you keep your juicer clean. Because of the type of foods, you'll be using, these machines require thorough scrubbing. Make sure you can get into all the nooks and crannies.

Ultimately, choose a juicer that makes things easy for you! This is the most important part of staying on track with your diet and feeling your best!

Why Investing in the Sirtfood Diet is Investing in Your Health

The cost of healthcare in America is high, and it is still rising. CNBC's article 'Here's How Much the Average American Spends on Health Care' cited data from the Centers for Medicare and Medicaid Services, noting that in 2016, Americans on average had to spend

$10,345 on healthcare compared to the $7,700 they spent for the same causes in 2007. That figure is forecast to steadily increase through the years, reaching a staggering $14,944 by 2023.

It is now imperative that you make an honest accounting of your health today, and if necessary, make the required changes that will ensure a healthier—and even wealthier—future. One aspect of your life that you may need to take a good, long look at is your diet.

A Diet for a Healthier You

Enter the Sirtfood Diet which promotes weight loss by activating the sirtuin pathways that impact metabolism, aging, and mood. These pathways are activated through the intake of polyphenol-rich foods referred to quite aptly as "sirtfoods." The Sirtfood Diet which is covered in-depth on our page 'The Sirtfood Diet is the Newest and Latest Strategy for Health, Nutrition and Weight Loss', offers a host of other health benefits, too, such as muscle building and memory enhancement.

One big advantage of the Sirtfood Diet is the effect it could have on your healthcare costs. Through following the diet you will get sick less often which in turn will require minimal health maintenance and monitoring. A healthier you, therefore, will no longer have to spend copious amounts on doctor's fees, medical procedures, and supplements. Some of the top sirtfoods to improve health and reduce costs include blueberries, strawberries, kale, chocolate (those of the 85% real cocoa variety only), citrus, coffee, and matcha green tea.

Lowered Costs on Health Insurance

A healthier you can also get comprehensive health insurance at very affordable rates. Lauren Gensler, in her article for Forbes, notes that the life insurance start-up Health IQ, founded by Like creator and highly regarded entrepreneur Munjal Shah, is quietly rewarding the health-conscious by offering inclusive insurance at lower premiums.

Shah's start-up, says Gensler, partners with established life insurance companies, and these partnerships allow Health IQ to offer health-conscious people (e.g. vegans, runners, yogis, and HITT practitioners) rates that are on average 4% to 33% lower than rates traditionally offered by other companies. Alex Rampell, a partner at Andreessen Horowitz and a resource for Gensler's article, believes this setup of offering lower rates to the health-conscious addresses a "fundamental unfairness of underwriting": those who mind their health are paying just as much as those who seemingly pay no heed to theirs.

A Venture Beat report, citing an interview with Shah, notes that the start-up is data-driven with an extensive, up-to-the-tiniest-of detail, documentation that allows the company to accurately identify people who deserve to be rewarded for living a healthy life – like those who follow healthy diets like the Sirtfood Diet or a vegan diet. Health IQ then helps these people get better insurance at lower premiums.

The perfect time to live a healthy life is always now, and adopting the Sirtfood Diet is most definitely a step in the right direction. Making this lifestyle change will lead to a healthier you, plus a bevy of other benefits in the other aspects of your life, including reducing your health costs.

Do You Need To Supplement The Sirtfood Diet?

Unless specifically prescribed for you by a medical or another health-care professional, a wide use of nutritional supplements is not recommended. With the Sirtfood Diet, you would be ingesting a vast and synergistic array of natural-plant compounds that provide the benefits. You cannot replicate these benefits with supplements and in fact, some in high doses may interfere with the beneficial effects of the Sirtfoods.

But are there any nutrients that fall short in the Sirtfood Diet that may need topping up? Whenever possible it is more advantageous to get the nutrients you need from eating a balanced diet rich in Sirtfoods, rather than in pill form. However, it is very difficult to get every single nutrient you need in optimum amounts, no matter how hard you try. The two nutrients you are likely to fall short of are Vitamin D (through the winter months) and selenium. Vegans will also have special nutritional considerations and these will be the subject of a later article.

Selenium-Supplement

What is it? Selenium is a trace mineral found in plants as well as some meat and seafood. The amount of selenium in foods is affected by how much selenium was in the soil they were grown in and how much the food has been processed.

Why do I need it? Selenium is essential for ridding the body of free radicals linked to premature aging and the development of chronic disease. In fact, recent research suggests that selenium deficiency may be a major factor in the rise of heart disease and cancer over the last few decades. Although we only need a small amount of selenium to be healthy, deficiencies in it are becoming more common, due to poor soil conditions and increased reliance on processed foods.

How do I get it? Good sources of selenium are brazil nuts, cashews, peanuts, eggs, alfalfa, mackerel, tuna, garlic, oysters, wholegrain cereals, and yeast.

The best way to supplement is in the form of selenium yeast and 50 to 100 mcg a day is recommended.

Vitamin D-Supplement

Vitamin D is a fat soluble vitamin that has a key role in helping calcium be absorbed in the gastrointestinal tract to support the growth and maintenance of our bones, as well as controlling calcium levels in the blood.

The signs for low vitamin D levels include low mood, feelings of fatigue, joint and muscle pain, and muscle weakness.

Low vitamin D levels has also been linked to a number of other health issues including neurological dysfunction, heart disease, diabetes, and some types of cancers although research into these associated disease states is in its early stages.

The biggest issue with low levels of vitamin D over time is that it puts our bone health at considerable risk. Low vitamin D results in high bone turnover, reduced bone density and an increased risk of fractures over time, especially in older people. While we can get vitamin D from a few specific foods including egg yolks, oily fish including sardines and salmon, fortified milks and some types of mushrooms, the amounts of vitamin D we get from food are relatively small, estimated at just 5-10 % of the total amount we require.

For this reason, sunshine is the primary source of vitamin D for most people. Vitamin D is produced in the body when our skin cells are exposed to ultraviolet B (UVB) light that we get from the sun.

And you don't need to sit in the sun for hours to get the amounts of vitamin D you need.

The average person will need between 5-10 minutes of sunlight exposure in Summer, versus up to 30 minutes in Winter, while darker skin types may require more. While we often expose our arms, larger parts of our body such as our chest, tummy or back will benefit from sun exposure thanks to their larger surface areas.

You cannot diagnose your own vitamin D deficiency. Rather you will need a blood test from your GP who will determine what your vitamin D levels are. Low levels of vitamin D can easily be fixed via an oral supplement which is best taken at night. It is important to know that there are two types of vitamin D, Vitamin D3 (cholecalciferol) is produced by the human body in response to sunlight compared to vitamin D2 (ergocalciferol) which is not produced in the human body, but is created by exposing certain plant-derived materials to ultraviolet light and is not as well absorbed in the body as Vitamin D3. So make sure you purchase Vitamin D3 if you do need a supplement.

Vitamin D deficiency is, therefore, a major concern, on a global scale, with research suggesting that nearly half the world's population may have less of this nutrient than they need.

Safe sun during the summer and a daily supplement of 1,000IU in the winter months will provide your vitamin needs.

SIRTFOOD COMPARED

We know that Sirtfoods and some other foods are good for us, whether its veggies like broccoli or tomatoes, spices like turmeric, or beverages like green tea. The reason these – and many other plant foods – are good for us, is primarily down to the bio-active plant compounds they contain. For the nutritionally savvy, we might be thinking of sulforaphane from broccoli, lycopene from tomatoes, curcumin from turmeric, and catechins from green tea. All the subject of extensive scientific research that goes a long way to explaining just why these foods are so good for our health.

But rather than just eating those individual foods, as good as they are, what if mixing certain foods – and therefore their nutrients – together at meals delivered an even bigger health boost? What if we could create synergies between nutrients in different foods that amplify their health benefits? It's a new idea, and here are a top-five of examples of how foods (and you will recognize the Sirtfoods in this list) can add up for maximum effect.

1. Green tea + lemon: Green tea drinkers can expect numerous health benefits given that consuming this prized beverage is linked with less cancer, heart disease, diabetes, and osteoporosis. These health benefits can be explained by its exceptional content of plant compounds called catechins, and especially a type called epigallocatechin gallate (EGCG). Adding a

squeeze of lemon juice to your green tea, which is rich in vitamin C, helps to significantly increase the number of catechins that get absorbed into the body.

2. Tomato sauce + extra virgin olive oil: Lycopene is the carotenoid responsible for the deep red color of tomatoes, and its consumption is linked with a reduced risk of certain cancers (most notably cancer of the prostate), cardiovascular disease, osteoporosis, and even protecting the skin from the damaging effects of the sun. The first thing to know about lycopene is that cooking and processing tomatoes dramatically increases the amount of lycopene that the body can absorb. The second is that the presence of fat further increases lycopene absorption. So teaming up your tomato-based dishes with a generous drizzle of extra virgin olive oil makes perfect sense.

3. Turmeric + black pepper: Turmeric, the bright yellow spice ever-present in traditional Indian cooking, is the subject of intense scientific study for its anti-cancer properties, it's potential to reduce inflammation in the body, and even for staving off dementia. This is believed to be primarily due to its active constituent curcumin. But the problem with curcumin is that it is very poorly absorbed by the body. However, adding black pepper increases its absorption, making them the perfect spice double-act. Cooking turmeric in liquid, and adding fat, further helps with curcumin absorption.

4. Broccoli + mustard: It's no secret that broccoli is good for us, with benefits including reducing cancer risk. Broccoli's main cancer-preventive ingredient is sulforaphane. This is formed when we eat broccoli by the action of an enzyme found in broccoli called myrosinase. However, cooking broccoli – especially over-cooking it – begins to destroy the myrosinase enzyme, reducing the amount of sulforaphane that can be made. In fact, if we're not careful, we can cook the benefits right out of broccoli. However, for those who like their broccoli well-cooked (rather than lightly steamed for 2 to 4 minutes), adding in other natural sources of myrosinase, such as from mustard or horseradish, means that sulforaphane can still be made.

5. Salad + avocado: Green leafy vegetables such as kale, spinach, and watercress, are packed full of health-promoting carotenoids such as immune-strengthening beta-carotene and eye-friendly lutein. However, when eaten raw, in the form of salads, these carotenoids are more difficult to absorb. But the addition of some fat can really help with that and adding avocado, rich in monounsaturated fat, to a salad, has been shown to dramatically increase the number of carotenoids that can be absorbed.

SUCCESS STORIES

FIRST STORY

What is it: The Sirtfood Diet, created by nutritionists Aidan Goggins and Glen Matten, and a favorite of trainer Pete Geracimo, who has all of his clients — Adele and Pippa Middleton included — follow the plan.

Who tried it: Julie Mazziotta, PEOPLE Writer/Reporter

Difficulty: 9/10 — So. Hungry. (At least for the first three days!)

In between racking up Grammy Awards, recording three hit albums, and becoming a mom, Adele has quietly slimmed down with the help of trainer Pete Geracimo. Under his instruction, the singer hits the gym (whether she wants to or not) and follows the Sirtfood Diet, which focuses on about 20 "wonder foods" like arugula, celery, cocoa, coffee, red onion and more.

I have no kids and a terrible singing voice, so testing out the diet for myself seemed like my only option to become more like Adele. Plus, dieters are clinically proven to lose 7 lbs. in the first seven days on the program, and I'd be A-Okay with that. So I gladly volunteered to try out week one.

Day 0:

Step one, before the diet actually started, was to read through The Sirtfood Diet and make a grocery list. On the first three days of the program, I would be slurping down three green juices — made up of kale, arugula, ginger, green apple, parsley, lemon, and matcha powder — and just one meal per day. This should have triggered a giant red flag for me, but the meals I did get sounded great — miso and sesame-glazed tofu with ginger and chili stir-fried greens, shrimp stir-fry with buckwheat noodles — plus after three days you go up to two meals a day, and two green juices. So I happily went off to Whole Foods.

The recipes thankfully are filled with ingredients you can find at any grocery store, anywhere in the country — except for one thing: buckwheat. I couldn't find it on my first shopping trip (the only reason why I went to Whole Foods for my groceries in the first place), and it took me another two tries to finally locate the grain (thanks, Chelsea Whole Foods!).

Buckwheat and the other sirtfoods are the focal points of the diet because they're high in polyphenols — a plant-based nutrient that Goggins and Matten say are great for the digestive system.

Polyphenols "activate a powerful recycling process in the body which clears out cellular waste and burns fat," the duo writes in the book. "They do this by activating our sirtuin genes — also known as our 'skinny' genes. Indeed, these are the very same genes that are activated by fasting and exercise."

Day 1:

That morning, perfectly content after enjoying my usual three (healthy-ish!) meals the day before, I cracked open my first green juice to start the diet (I will admit here that I cheated a bit from the start — I don't have a juicer, nor the space in my apartment to store one, so I bought juices that matched the ingredients in Sirtfood's recipe from Juice Press and Pressed Juicery in New York City). Pretty good! I've never been a regular green juice-drinker, but this was enjoyable enough.

I kept sipping throughout the day and started getting my usual hunger calls around 11 a.m. I have a pretty severe snack addiction, but I at least go for the healthy stuff, like pistachios and granola bars, and this was normally when I get my fix. But I pushed through. Goggins and Matten say that you can eat your one meal at any time of the day, so I decided to go for 4 p.m.

By 1 p.m., I was miserable and starving. The green juice did absolutely nothing to curb my hunger, which makes sense — nothing in it has real staying power. I regularly write the What I Eat columns, and I kept thinking about the nutritionists who talk about the need for meals with protein to keep you satisfied, something I was severely lacking. My day piled up, so I somehow didn't actually eat until 5 p.m. Luckily, the meal was DELICIOUS. I went for the aforementioned miso-glazed tofu, and I would make this any day of the week. I even managed to save part of it to eat when I got home from work as a "dinner" (is it against the rules to split up the one meal? I was too hungry to care).

Day 2:

More green juice. More hunger.

Today's meal was harissa-baked tofu with cauliflower "couscous." I'm not vegetarian, but I'm not a big fan of shrimp, the other option that day. I probably should have gone with it anyway though — this meal was a big miss for me. It again lacked anything satisfying, so I was miserable the entire day, particularly when I somberly followed my friends to dinner at Sweetgreen (probably my all-time favorite fast-casual restaurant) that night and sipped the ubiquitous green juice as they munched on salads. Yes, I was jealous of salads.

Day 3:

You guessed it! I had green juice for breakfast.

My meal today was kale and red onion dal with buckwheat, and WOW. I loved it. I wanted piles of it. But my one portion was surprisingly satisfying — I think at this point my appetite had gone down from eating under 1,000 calories a day, plus the dal included plenty of satiating ingredients, like lentils, buckwheat (I found it!) and healthy fat-filled coconut milk. I don't weigh myself, but by day three I was comfortably wearing my tightest pair of skinny jeans, and my normally rounded stomach was much flatter.

The only remaining problem? I'm someone who exercises regularly, and hard. I go to CrossFit three times a week, sometimes more, and I run or swim on the other days. With such a low-calorie count that wasn't recommended (I emailed Goggins, who said,

"The mild calorie restriction plus the high intake of sirtuin-activating nutrients is creating a mild stress on our cells which causes sirtuin activity to strongly kick in. Too much exercise just causes too much stress, which could then be detrimental"), but I love the head-clearing benefits of exercise. I went to CrossFit that night, and knowing I wanted to go again in the morning for the usual Saturday workout, I hard-boiled two eggs and ate them with Old Bay and drizzled extra-virgin olive oil, my favorite. It was beyond necessary.

Day 4:

I could finally eat two meals a day — hooray! But my tough workout unsurprisingly didn't go well on such little food over the last three days. So with the increase in food on the plan, I decided to switch things up — I would go back to eating normally and just try out the other recipes for the rest of the week. I'm stubborn and highly competitive, so it was frustrating to "fail" at the diet, but I also really, really love food, and skipping one to two meals a day was not worth it to me.

The rest of the week:

The other meals I tried — pan-fried salmon with caramelized endive, arugula and celery leaf salad (it also has avocado!); Tuscan bean stew; the sirt super salad; the sirtfood omelet — were all similarly fantastic. I want to give a hearty props to Goggins and Matten for crafting recipes that are delicious and filled with normal ingredients — plus they were often one-pan meals, which is key for someone without a dishwasher nor a person to do the dishes for you (which I'm of course assuming Adele has — livin' the dream).

The Verdict:

If you are immune to hunger and really enjoy green juices, go for it (and check with your doctor beforehand)! If you're more like me, skip week one, and go straight to week two, when you get to enjoy three full and truly excellent meals a day. And you can still pretend to be Adele.

SECOND STORY

What It Is: Crossrope, an at-home jump rope workout

Who Tried It: Stephanie Emma Pfeffer, PEOPLE Health writer, and editor

Level of Difficulty: 5

You know those people who are working out more than ever right now because they have so much extra time?

I envy them. Pre-pandemic, I worked out when my kids were at school. Now that they're with me 24/7, I've had to get creative with exercise.

Usually, I run. But since this whole thing started, I've had more races canceled than opportunities to get out there. While I have made meager attempts to cruise around the neighborhood pushing my 4-year-old in the BOB stroller while simultaneously (!) pulling my 7-

year-old on her scooter, it's Not. The. Same. I would give anything for a child-free, uninterrupted 12-miler these days.

For me, exercise is as much a physical thing as it is mental. It helps regulate my moods and enables me to be more patient with my kids. Unfortunately, this is a time when I need more patience than ever, but there are few ways to get it. Sure, I have done a bunch of at-home workouts, but what I was really missing was endorphin-boosting cardio.

So when I heard about Crossrope, I was intrigued. I had actually been using a speed rope at home on and off, but getting this kit made a big difference in my routine. First, the ropes are weighted — the "Get Lean" bundle comes with 1/4-lb. and 1/2-lb. ropes for $99 — which made for a smooth and fluid swing and no twisty, tangled-up ropes. There's also a "Get Strong" bundle ($139) for more muscle activation that comes with 1- and 2-lb. ropes.

What makes this convenient is that jump rope can be done in relatively small spaces. I put a yoga mat in the corner of my bedroom to protect my floor (and my neighbors) and was pleased to discover that even mid-jump, my rope cleared the ceiling.

Crossrope's free app offers a bunch of useful workouts. They range from beginner to advanced, from endurance to HIIT — and the ones I tried felt manageable and fun. My favorites incorporated bodyweight exercises into the routine; for example, 60 seconds of freestyle jump followed by 30 seconds of burpees and then 30 seconds of rest.

Other workouts alternated between jump and rest intervals, although during the rest periods I would usually grab my dumbbells or do core work. Again, my ropes were the lightest offered — I'd probably take more advantage of the rest periods if using heavier ropes that fired up even more muscle groups. There's also an active Facebook community that I found to be inspiring, supportive, and full of cool tips.

One of my favorite aspects of this workout is that it allowed me to stop and start a million times for kid interruptions. The intervals were short, so I could always tell my kids "15 more seconds," or even pause mid-workout to disseminate snacks before getting back to it. But I also liked how, whenever I had just a few free minutes throughout the day, I could grab the ropes and get my heart rate up. I didn't need a 50-minute window to make it happen. In that respect, it was even a tiny bit more convenient than running.

On average I burned about 250+ calories per 25-minute workout, which helped me feel like I was not the laziest person on earth. This was just doing basic, quick jumps, so I definitely have room to improve. (And learn tricks!)

The Verdict: This is an awesome quarantine workout option. You could probably even lose a few pounds if you were not baking banana bread, eating your feelings, and being crushed by two tiny humans depending on you for every homeschool lesson, meal, bath, a moment of entertainment, arts-and-crafts idea, etc. At least Crossrope will help me keep the "quarantine 15" at bay while ensuring that I don't completely lose my fitness — or my mind.

THIRD STORY

What It Is: A session at TB12, Tom Brady's sports therapy center in Foxborough, MA

Who Tried It: Stephanie Emma Pfeffer, PEOPLE Health writer, and editor

Level of Difficulty: 4/10 — The treatment is highly individualized and depends on your performance goals and/or injuries. That said, the deep tissue massage can be beastly if your muscles are tight!

A partnership between Tom Brady and his longtime trainer and business partner Alex Guerrero, TB12 first opened six years ago in the shadow of Gillette Stadium, home of the New England Patriots. The sports therapy center helps top athletes not only recover from injuries (rehab) but also prevent them (known as pre-hab). The body coaches practice Guerrero's legendary methods of helping people achieve peak athletic performance using functional training that mimics what they actually do on the field, court, etc. At the core is a holistic approach to health.

When I first walked in, I couldn't believe how small it was. This is where legends train? It's about 6,000-sq. feet of open space covered by turf on one half of the main floor and maybe six high-tech cardio machines on the other half, plus a basketball hoop. Not a free weight insight. The space is flanked by eight private rooms with sports massage tables.

I expected an intimidating atmosphere but my body coach Matt Denning — who has his doctorate in physical therapy and trained under Guerrero himself — put me at ease as he asked about my athletic history. A runner, I came in sore, having just completed a hilly half marathon. I admitted that even before the race my lower back had been hurting, so Denning made easing that pain one of our primary goals.

Deep-Force Muscle Pliability Work

We went into one of the side rooms to start the deep tissue work, which felt like a painful massage. He started with the bottom of my feet (I apologized profusely for not having gotten a pedicure — I didn't know!), which were extremely tight from running.

As he continued to work on my legs, Denning explained that my hip flexor seemed to be carrying too much of my running load, which should be more evenly distributed into my glutes. "The glute is our biggest and strongest muscle so you need to be efficient with that," he said, adding that my lower back pain was likely from tight muscles overloading the joints and ligaments.

This was one of the pliability components of our session (the other was at the end when we used a vibrating foam roller). I was skeptical when I first heard the term pliability. I mean, isn't that the same as flexibility? I stretch post-run — do I need to do more? Actually, yes. I learned pliability helps in injury prevention. "It's not how long the muscles are, but how soft that tissue is, how effective that tissue is," Denning said. "When you have pliable tissue, it's more vascular, there is better blood flow, it's more efficient, it can fully relax and contract. When not pliable, the tissue is tight, so when there is trauma, like getting hit in football or running a hard race, that load will be transferred to a joint or a ligament." In short, pliability aids in recovery.

Hydration and Nutrition

During the deep tissue work, we talked a lot about the center's multi-faceted approach, including hydration and nutrition. Denning recommends drinking half your body weight in ounces each day. "Our muscles are 80 percent water, so we need to be sufficiently hydrated so we can do all the metabolic functions they need to and make the necessary nerve connections," he said.

Asked what I eat, I told him I start the day with a plant-based protein shake — Brady has his own line of TB12 protein powder — and then I might have an egg on avocado toast for lunch. I snack on peanut butter and yogurt and fruit but admitted that dinner is tricky at my house with two young, picky kids. Denning recommended a few simple changes: I should stay away from foods that have inflammatory properties, like peanuts. That means swapping peanut butter for almond butter (and if I do want PB, never before a race). He also suggested I reduce my dairy intake. "Limiting how much inflammation is systemically in our body helps us recover, so if you have a tough run, your quads shouldn't be as sore if you remove the inflammation already in the body."

But above all, he encouraged moderation. "We don't expect everyone to eat exactly as Tom does," said Denning, alluding to Brady's restrictive mostly plant-based, dairy-free, gluten-free, sugar-free, white flour-free, caffeine-free and alcohol-free (you get the idea) diet. "Most 42-year olds don't have to get hit by 300-lb. people, that's not everyone's daily life."

And how often does the famous quarterback swing by? "During the [football] season, he's here a lot because he's getting more load on his body, and also because of the proximity of the center to the stadium," Denning said. "In the offseason — when he's not traveling or doing stuff with the family — he's in a couple of times a week."

His wife Gisele Bündchen is no stranger to TB12, either. Denning said she comes in very often. "She will work with one of our body coaches a couple of times a week for most of the year," he said. "She's one of the hardest workers here. She's got great form." Apparently, she's there so much that she has her own reserve of TB12 protein powder — the bag is marked with a big "G."

Functional Strength and Conditioning

After Denning finished the deep tissue work, we went to the floor machines, which included an anti-gravity treadmill. This particular one came from Brady's house — he used it to accelerate his recovery after he blew out his ACL in 2008. This is one cool machine: By reducing an athlete's body weight (it can go as low as 20 percent!), it allows them to get back to moving more quickly and reinforces the neuropathways that improve muscle memory. I was zipped into what looked like a plastic skirt with spandex shorts before an air compressor essentially sucked out the gravity and made me feel like I was running on air. There was virtually no impact on my joints, so I totally understood how it could physically and psychologically help a sidelined athlete recover faster.

This anti-gravity treadmill is the one Tom Brady had in his house while recovering from his torn ACL in 2008.

Denning also analyzed my gait, which I was pleased to learn was pretty even on my left and right sides. (One less thing to worry about!) But although my walking and running were symmetrical, he again said I appear to be quad and hip-flexor dominant, so my glutes aren't stabilizing my pelvis, which might be contributing to my lower back pain. It could even be negatively impacting my running times since I am essentially not using the biggest muscle in my body as efficiently as I could be.

That theme continued as I tried a self-propelled TrueForm treadmill. Denning explained that with a lot of motorized treadmills since you're not generating ground force — just picking up your legs — running becomes more of a hip flexor activity. But with this machine, because you have to propel the treadmill forward, it keeps your biomechanics neutral (spine neutral versus flexed forward) and forces the power to come from your glutes. I realized that all of my race training had been happening on indoor treadmills during the winter, which might be why my glutes were weak. I vowed to train outdoors more often now that the weather is warm.

The TruForm treadmill was also covered in turf so athletes can run on it in their cleats. Denning said that almost everything done at TB12 is intended to mimic an athlete's true movement and experience. That's why there are no free weights. Everything is about body weight, pliability work or dynamic warmup to activate tissue for functional training.

Next up we did some strengthening exercises on the turf, which was again, very specific to my goals as a runner. We focused on the single-leg stance for the stability of my hips, followed by resistance band squats, planks, and a glute med side plank. Everything was also high intensity, like a circuit.

"When we do this at high intensity, it helps boost testosterone levels and eliminate cortisol production so we can burn belly fat and build the muscle," he said. "We want to load up your muscles with good resistance, but it's not going to your joints like traditional weight lifting."

While TB12 is a haven for athletes, it services all types of clients. Denning says the youngest is a 3-year-old girl with an injury from birth, while the oldest is a man in his mid-80s. "And we have everything in between," he says. "Some people come for performance enhancement, or to experience what Tom experiences, or for rehab, maybe post-op. We have all ages and pathologies."

And now more people will have the chance to try it out. A second TB12 location is set to open in early August in a much more central and highly trafficked location, Boston's Back Bay neighborhood. At 10,000-sq. feet, it will be almost double the size of the Foxborough center, which is 30 miles southwest of the city.

Boston's new TB12, which happens to be near the finish line of the Boston Marathon, will also include a group fitness studio, which will probably make it more accessible to the public. (Currently, only one-on-one sessions are available, and they cost around $200.)"From the beginning, Alex and Tom have wanted to help as many people as possible," says Denning. "This new location will allow them to do that."

The Verdict: For serious athletes, a person recovering from an injury or anyone with a specific performance goal in mind, a visit to TB12 can increase awareness of weakness, asymmetry, or problem areas and give you tangible, functional ways to improve. It will be even more accessible — both in location and cost — when the Boston outpost opens this summer.

FORTH STORY

What It Is: The Empire State Building Run-Up, the world's first — and most famous — tower race

Who Tried It: Stephanie Emma Pfeffer, PEOPLE Health writer, and editor

Level of Difficulty: 8/10 — Thigh burning, lung-bursting... but with a great payoff at the top.

When PEOPLE got an invitation to participate in the Empire State Building Run-Up sponsored by Turkish Airlines (which is headquartered there), I knew I couldn't pass up the opportunity to do one of the most iconic races in the world, one that benefits charities like the Challenged Athletes Foundation and the Multiple Myeloma Research Foundation.

While I was pretty sure I would be able to make it to the top, I knew it was a different beast than my usual half-marathons: I needed to be quick and powerful versus slow(er) and steady. About a month out, I increased my HIIT workouts and threw in a few extra split squats and lunges. (Obviously, I'm not a trainer — I just guessed what might make sense.) I also used the StairMaster at the gym several times a week, figuring the Empire State Building setting would totally prepare me for the thigh burn.

Not quite! It was still a challenge. The first 20 floors were easy enough, but then I started feeling it in my chest and lungs. The stairs are also pretty steep. I remember reaching the halfway point and thinking, wow, my quads are already kind of tired and I have another 40 floors to go! So no, it wasn't really like the StairMaster — but that training probably helped my endurance.

And 17 minutes after entering the stairwell, I blew through the door of the 86th floor and literally felt on top of the world! Since the runners are staggered, there are just a few finishers at a time. It was really cool to be on the 86th floor of the Empire State Building — usually teeming with tourists — with just a handful of other people. I felt special for a few seconds... before heading all the way back down in the elevator.

Here's what else I learned climbing 86 flights, 1,576 stairs, approximately one-fifth of a vertical mile to the top:

Double up! It was most efficient to take two steps at a time. But I did switch to single steps periodically when my quads needed a break from the exertion.

Handrails help. The stairwell was narrow enough to grab the rails on both sides and use them to pull yourself up for momentum. It's legal in this race and is one of the main tips given by elite runners.

Dust is not your friend. The worst part for me was the burning in my throat, presumably caused by my rapid breathing + a dusty, enclosed space. The two water stations helped but my throat still hurt 10 minutes post-climb.

It was not crowded at all! Not only were the heats staggered (elite, charity runners, media, etc.), but each person entered the stairs 5 seconds after the person before. I'd expected a massive cluster of people trying to elbow each other out of the way. But there was plenty of space, and runners were nice to each other, stepping aside if someone was trying to pass, but also asking: "Are you OK? Hang in there!"

Tower running is a thing. There are tower run clubs all over the world, and running enthusiasts work the tower run circuit, traveling from city to city to compete.

It's super exclusive. The race had just 217 finishers. I met one woman who said she had tried to get in via lottery for the past 10 years!

The payoff on the 86th floor was completely worth it. There is no way to describe the exhilaration that comes with the view, the realization of what you've accomplished — and the fact that you are standing on top of the greatest city in the world.

The fastest runner was a 33-year-old from Poland who finished in 10:05. The next group of elite runners didn't finish until at least a minute later. My finishing time of 17:28 placed me sixth in my age group. The last finisher was an 81-year-old man. That guy is my hero!

THE DIET PLANNING PHASES

The plan claims that eating certain foods will activate your "skinny gene" pathway and have you losing seven pounds in seven days. Foods like kale, dark chocolate, and wine contain a natural chemical called polyphenols that mimic the effects of exercise and fasting. Strawberries, red onions, cinnamon, and turmeric are also powerful sirtfoods. These foods will trigger the sirtuin pathway to help trigger weight loss. The science sounds enticing, but in reality, there's little research to back up these claims. Plus, the promised rate of weight loss in the first week is rather quick and not in line with the National Institute of Health safe weight loss guidelines of one to two pounds per week.

The diet has two phases:

· Phase 1 lasts for seven days. For the first three days, you drink three sirtfood green juices and one meal rich in sirtfoods for a total of 1,000 calories. On days four through seven, you drink two green juices and two meals for a total of 1,500 calories.

· Phase 2 is a 14-day maintenance plan, although it is designed for you to lose weight steadily (not maintain your current weight). Each day consists of three balanced sirtfood meals and one green juice.

After these three weeks, you're encouraged to continue eating a diet rich in sirtfoods and drinking a green juice daily. You can find several sirtfood cookbooks online and recipes on the sirtfood website. One green juice recipe found on the sirtfood website consists of a combo of kale and other leafy greens, parsley, celery, green apple, ginger, lemon juice, and matcha. Buckwheat and lovage are also ingredients that are recommended for use in your green juice. The diet recommends that juices should be made in a juicer, not a blender, so it tastes better.

A day on the sirtfood diet might look like this:

Breakfast: Soy yogurt with mixed berries, chopped walnuts, and dark chocolate

Lunch: A sirtfood salad made with kale, parsley, celery, apple, walnuts topped with olive oil mixed with lemon juice and ginger.

Dinner: Stir-fried prawns with kale and buckwheat noodles.

*Plus one sirtfood green juice per day.

The Costs

You really need to plan and have access to the recommended ingredients in order to properly follow this diet. You'll also need to invest in a decent juicer, which can cost you a minimum of $100. Besides the free recipes available on the website, you may need to invest in some of The Sirtfood Diet cookbooks.

The seasonality of ingredients makes it a bit tough to get strawberries and kale certain times of the year. It's also tough to follow when traveling, at social events, and feeding a family with young kids.

The diet itself cuts out numerous food groups and is limiting. Dairy foods, which provide an array of essential nutrients including several that most folks lack, aren't recommended on the plan. Further, the polyphenol-rich food matcha often contains lead in the tea leaves which is potentially dangerous to your health especially when taken regularly. It also has a strong and bitter flavor, as does 85% dark chocolate, which is also recommended.

The Bottom Line: Polyphenol-rich foods can certainly be included in a weight loss plan, but they aren't the basis for an entire diet. You most certainly don't need wine and dark chocolate every day, plus too much matcha is potentially dangerous.

BENEFITS

There is growing evidence that sirtuin activators may have a wide range of health benefits as well as building muscle and suppressing appetite. These include improving memory, helping the body better control blood sugar levels, and cleaning up the damage from free radical molecules that can accumulate in cells and lead to cancer and other diseases.

'Substantial observational evidence exists for the beneficial effects of the intake of food and drinks rich in sirtuin activators in decreasing risks of chronic disease,' said Professor Frank Hu, an expert in nutrition and epidemiology at Harvard University in a recent article in the journal Advances In Nutrition. A sirtfood diet is particularly suitable as an anti-aging regime.

Although sirtuin activators are found all through the plant kingdom, only certain fruits and vegetables have large enough amounts to counting as sirtfoods. Examples include green tea, cocoa powder, the Indian spice turmeric, kale, onions, and parsley.

Many of the fruit and vegetables on display in supermarkets, such as tomatoes, avocados, bananas, lettuce, kiwis, carrots, and cucumber, are actually rather low in sirtuin activators. This doesn't mean that they aren't worth eating, though, as they provide lots of other benefits.

The beauty of eating a diet packed with sirtfoods is that it's far more flexible than other diets. You could simply eat healthily adding some sirtfoods on top. Or you could have them in a concentrated way. Adding sirtfoods to say, the 5:2 diet could allow more calories on the low-calorie days.

A remarkable finding of one sirtfood diet trial is that participants lost substantial weight without losing muscle. In fact, it was common for participants to actually gain muscle, leading to a more defined and toned look. That's the beauty of sirtfoods; they activate fat burning but also promote muscle growth, maintenance, and repair. This is in complete contrast to other diets where weight loss typically comes from both fat and muscle, with the loss of muscle slowing down metabolism and making weight regain more likely.

RECIPES FOR YOU

TURMERIC CHICKEN & KALE SALAD WITH HONEY LIME DRESSING

Prep Time: 20mins

Cook Time: 10mins

Serves: 2

Ingredients

For the chicken

1 teaspoon ghee or 1 tbsp coconut oil

½ medium brown onion, diced

250-300 g / 9 oz. chicken mince or diced up chicken thighs

1 large garlic clove, finely diced

1 teaspoon turmeric powder

1teaspoon lime zest

juice of ½ lime

½ teaspoon salt + pepper

For the salad

6 broccolini stalks or 2 cups of broccoli florets

2 tablespoons pumpkin seeds (pepitas)

3 large kale leaves, stems removed and chopped

½ avocado, sliced

handful of fresh coriander leaves, chopped

handful of fresh parsley leaves, chopped

For the dressing

3 tablespoons lime juice

1 small garlic clove, finely diced or grated

3 tablespoons extra-virgin olive oil

1 teaspoon raw honey

½ teaspoon wholegrain or Dijon mustard

½ teaspoon sea salt and pepper

Instructions

1. Heat the ghee or coconut oil in a small frying pan over medium-high heat. Add the onion and sauté on medium heat for 4-5 minutes, until golden. Add the chicken mince and garlic and stir for 2-3 minutes over medium-high heat, breaking it apart.

2. Add the turmeric, lime zest, lime juice, salt and pepper and cook, stirring frequently, for a further 3-4 minutes. Set the cooked mince aside.

3. While the chicken is cooking, bring a small saucepan of water to boil. Add the broccolini and cook for 2

minutes. Rinse under cold water and cut into 3-4 pieces each.

4. Add the pumpkin seeds to the frying pan from the chicken and toast over medium heat for 2 minutes, stirring frequently to prevent burning. Season with a little salt. Set aside. Raw pumpkin seeds are also fine to use.

5. Place chopped kale in a salad bowl and pour over the dressing. Using your hands, toss and massage the kale with the dressing. This will soften the kale, kind of like what citrus juice does to fish or beef carpaccio – it 'cooks' it slightly.

6. Finally toss through the cooked chicken, broccolini, fresh herbs, pumpkin seeds and avocado slices.

RASPBERRY AND BLACKCURRANT JELLY

Ready in 15 minutes + setting time

Serves 2

Ingredients

100g raspberries, washed

2 leaves gelatine

100g blackcurrants, washed and stalks removed

2 tbsp granulated sugar

300ml water

Instructions

1. Arrange the raspberries in two serving dishes/glasses/moulds. Put the gelatine leaves in a bowl of cold water to soften.

2. Place the blackcurrants in a small pan with the sugar and 100ml water and bring to the boil. Simmer vigorously for 5 minutes and then remove from the heat. Leave to stand for 2 minutes.

3. Squeeze out excess water from the gelatine leaves and add them to the saucepan. Stir until fully dissolved, then stir in the rest of the water. Pour the liquid into the prepared dishes and refrigerate to set. The jellies should be ready in about 3-4 hours or overnight.

BUCKWHEAT NOODLES WITH CHICKEN KALE & MISO DRESSING

Prep Time: 15 mins

Cook Time: 15 mins

Serves: 2

Ingredients

For the noodles

2-3 handfuls of kale leaves (removed from the stem and roughly cut)

150 g / 5 oz buckwheat noodles (100% buckwheat, no wheat)

3-4 shiitake mushrooms, sliced

1 teaspoon coconut oil or ghee

1 brown onion, finely diced

1 medium free-range chicken breast, sliced or diced

1 long red chilli, thinly sliced (seeds in or out depending on how hot you like it)

2 large garlic cloves, finely diced

2-3 tablespoons Tamari sauce (gluten-free soy sauce)

For the miso dressing

1½ tablespoon fresh organic miso

1 tablespoon Tamari sauce

1 tablespoon extra-virgin olive oil

1 tablespoon lemon or lime juice

1 teaspoon sesame oil (optional)

Instructions

1. Bring a medium saucepan of water to boil. Add the kale and cook for 1 minute, until slightly wilted. Remove and set aside but reserve the water and bring it back to the boil. Add the soba noodles and cook according to the package instructions (usually about 5 minutes). Rinse under cold water and set aside.

2. In the meantime, pan fry the shiitake mushrooms in a little ghee or coconut oil (about a teaspoon) for 2-3 minutes, until lightly browned on each side. Sprinkle with sea salt and set aside.

3. In the same frying pan, heat more coconut oil or ghee over medium-high heat. Sauté onion and chilli for 2-3 minutes and then add the chicken pieces. Cook 5 minutes over medium heat, stirring a couple of times, then add the garlic, tamari sauce and a little splash of water. Cook for a further 2-3 minutes, stirring frequently until chicken is cooked through.

4. Finally, add the kale and soba noodles and toss through the chicken to warm up.

5. Mix the miso dressing and drizzle over the noodles right at the end of cooking, this way you will keep all those beneficial probiotics in the miso alive and active.

ASIAN KING PRAWN STIR-FRY WITH BUCKWHEAT NOODLES

Prep Time: 10mins

Cook Time: 10mins

Serves 1

Ingredients

150g shelled raw king prawns, deveined

2 tsp tamari (you can use soy sauce if you are not avoiding gluten)

2 tsp extra virgin olive oil

75g soba (buckwheat noodles)

1 garlic clove, finely chopped

1 bird's eye chilli, finely chopped

1 tsp finely chopped fresh ginger

20g red onions, sliced

40g celery, trimmed and sliced

75g green beans, chopped

50g kale, roughly chopped

100ml chicken stock

5g lovage or celery leaves

Instructions

1. Heat a frying pan over a high heat, then cook the prawns in 1 teaspoon of the tamari and 1 teaspoon of the oil for 2–3 minutes. Transfer the prawns to a plate. Wipe the pan out with kitchen paper, as you're going to use it again.

2. Cook the noodles in boiling water for 5–8 minutes or as directed on the packet. Drain and set aside.

3. Meanwhile, fry the garlic, chilli and ginger, red onion, celery, beans and kale in the remaining oil over a medium–high heat for 2–3 minutes. Add the stock and bring to the boil, then simmer for a minute or two, until the vegetables are cooked but still crunchy.

4. Add the prawns, noodles and lovage/celery leaves to the pan, bring back to the boil then remove from the heat and serve.

BAKED SALMON SALAD WITH CREAMY MINT DRESSING

Prep Time; 20mins

Serves 1

Ingredients

1 salmon fillet (130g)

40g mixed salad leaves

40g young spinach leaves

2 radishes, trimmed and thinly sliced

5cm piece (50g) cucumber, cut into chunks

2 spring onions, trimmed and sliced

1 small handful (10g) parsley, roughly chopped

For the dressing:

1 tsp low-fat mayonnaise

1 tbsp natural yogurt

1 tbsp rice vinegar

2 leaves mint, finely chopped

Salt and freshly ground black pepper

Instructions

1. Preheat the oven to 200°C (180°C fan/Gas 6).

2. Place the salmon fillet on a baking tray and bake for 16–18 minutes until just cooked through. Remove from the oven and set aside. The salmon is equally nice hot or cold in the salad. If your salmon has skin, simply cook skin side down and remove the salmon from the skin using a fish slice after cooking. It should slide off easily when cooked.

3. In a small bowl, mix together the mayonnaise, yogurt, rice wine vinegar, mint leaves and salt and pepper together and leave to stand for at least 5 minutes to allow the

flavors to develop.

4. Arrange the salad leaves and spinach on a serving plate and top with the radishes, cucumber, spring onions and parsley. Flake the cooked salmon onto the salad and drizzle the dressing over.

CHOC CHIP GRANOLA

Prep Time: 20mins

Cook Time: 10mins

Serves 8

Ingredients

200g jumbo oats

50g pecans, roughly chopped

3 tbsp light olive oil

20g butter

1 tbsp dark brown sugar

2 tbsp rice malt syrup

60g good-quality (70%)

dark chocolate chips

Instructions

1. Preheat the oven to 160°C (140°C fan/Gas 3). Line a large baking tray with a silicone sheet or baking parchment.

2. Mix the oats and pecans together in a large bowl. In a small non-stick pan, gently heat the olive oil, butter, brown sugar and rice malt syrup until the butter has melted and the sugar and syrup have dissolved. Do not

allow to boil. Pour the syrup over the oats and stir thoroughly until the oats are fully covered.

3. Distribute the granola over the baking tray, spreading right into the corners. Leave clumps of mixture with spacing rather than an even spread. Bake in the oven for 20 minutes until just tinged golden brown at the edges. Remove from the oven and leave to cool on the tray completely.

4. When cool, break up any bigger lumps on the tray with your fingers and then mix in the chocolate chips. Scoop or pour the granola into an airtight tub or jar. The granola will keep for at least 2 weeks.

FRAGRANT ASIAN HOTPOT

Prep Time: 5mins

Cook Time: 10mins

Serves 2

Ingredients

1 tsp tomato purée

1 star anise, crushed (or 1/4 tsp ground anise)

Small handful (10g) parsley, stalks finely chopped

Small handful (10g) coriander, stalks finely chopped

Juice of 1/2 lime

500ml chicken stock, fresh or made with 1 cube

1/2 carrot, peeled and cut into matchsticks

50g broccoli, cut into small florets

50g beansprouts

100g raw tiger prawns

100g firm tofu, chopped

50g rice noodles, cooked according to packet instructions

50g cooked water chestnuts, drained

20g sushi ginger, chopped

1 tbsp good-quality miso paste

Instructions

1. Place the tomato purée, star anise, parsley stalks, coriander stalks, lime juice and chicken stock in a large pan and bring to a simmer for 10 minutes.

2. Add the carrot, broccoli, prawns, tofu, noodles and water chestnuts and simmer gently until the prawns are cooked through. Remove from the heat and stir in the sushi ginger and miso paste.

3. Serve sprinkled with the parsley and coriander leaves.

LAMB,BUTTERNUT SQUASH AND DATE TAGINE

Prep Time: 15 mins

Cook Time: 1 hour 15 mins

Serves 4

Ingredients

2 tablespoons olive oil

1 red onion, sliced

2cm ginger, grated

3 garlic cloves, grated or crushed

1 teaspoon chilli flakes (or to taste)

2 teaspoons cumin seeds

1 cinnamon stick

2 teaspoons ground turmeric

800g lamb neck fillet, cut into 2cm chunks

½ teaspoon salt

100g medjool dates, pitted and chopped

400g tin chopped tomatoes, plus half a can of water

500g butternut squash, chopped into 1cm cubes

400g tin chickpeas, drained

2 tablespoons fresh coriander (plus extra for garnish)

Buckwheat, couscous, flatbreads or rice to serve

Instructions

1.Preheat your oven to 140C.

2.Drizzle about 2 tablespoons of olive oil into a large ovenproof saucepan or cast iron casserole dish. Add the sliced onion and cook on a gentle heat, with the lid on, for about 5 minutes, until the onions are softened but not brown.

3.Add the grated garlic and ginger, chilli, cumin, cinnamon and turmeric. Stir well and cook for 1 more minute with the lid off. Add a splash of water if it gets too dry.

4.Next add in the lamb chunks. Stir well to coat the meat in the onions and spices and then add the salt, chopped dates and tomatoes, plus about half a can of water (100-200ml).

5.Bring the tagine to the boil and then put the lid on and put in your preheated oven for 1 hour and 15 minutes.

6.Thirty minutes before the end of the cooking time, add in the chopped butternut squash and drained chickpeas. Stir everything together, put the lid back on and return to the oven for the final 30 minutes of cooking.

7.When the tagine is ready, remove from the oven and stir through the chopped coriander. Serve with buckwheat, couscous, flatbreads or basmati rice.

Notes

If you don't own an ovenproof saucepan or cast iron casserole dish, simply cook the tagine in a regular saucepan up until it has to go in the oven and then transfer the tagine into a regular lidded casserole dish before placing in the oven. Add on an extra 5 minutes cooking time to allow for the fact that the casserole dish will need extra time to heat up.

SIRTFOOD MUSHROOM SCRAMBLE EGGS

Ingredients

2 eggs

1 tsp ground turmeric

1 tsp mild curry powder

20g kale, roughly chopped

1 tsp extra virgin olive oil

½ bird's eye chilli, thinly sliced

handful of button mushrooms, thinly sliced

5g parsley, finely chopped

optional Add a seed mixture as a topper and some Rooster Sauce for flavor

Instructions

1. Mix the turmeric and curry powder and add a little water until you have achieved a light paste.

2. Steam the kale for 2– 3 minutes.

3. Heat the oil in a frying pan over a medium heat and fry the chilli and mushrooms for 2– 3 minutes until they have started to brown and soften.

PRAWN ARRABBIATA

Serves 1

Preparation time:

35 – 40 minutes

Cooking time:

20 – 30 minutes

Ingredients

125-150 g Raw or cooked prawns (Ideally king prawns)

65 g Buckwheat pasta

1 tbsp Extra virgin olive oil

For arrabbiata sauce

40 g Red onion, finely chopped

1 Garlic clove, finely chopped

30 g Celery, finely chopped

1 Bird's eye chilli, finely chopped

1 tsp Dried mixed herbs

1 tsp Extra virgin olive oil

2 tbsp White wine (optional)

400 g Tinned chopped tomatoes

1 tbsp Chopped parsley

Instructions

1. Fry the onion, garlic, celery and chilli and dried herbs in the oil over a medium–low heat for 1–2 minutes. Turn the heat up to medium, add the wine and cook for 1 minute. Add the tomatoes and leave the sauce to simmer over a medium–low heat for 20–30 minutes, until it has a nice rich consistency. If you feel the sauce is getting too thick simply add a little water.

2. While the sauce is cooking bring a pan of water to the boil and cook the pasta according to the packet instructions. When cooked to your liking, drain, toss with the olive oil and keep in the pan until needed.

3. If you are using raw prawns add them to the sauce and cook for a further 3–4 minutes, until they have turned pink and opaque, add the parsley and serve. If you are using cooked prawns add them with the parsley, bring the sauce to the boil and serve.

4. Add the cooked pasta to the sauce, mix thoroughly but gently and serve.

TURMERIC BAKED SALMON-SIRTFOOD RECIPES

Prep Time: 10 – 15 minutes

Cooking time: 10 minutes

Serves 1

Ingredients

125-150 g Skinned Salmon

1 tsp Extra virgin olive oil

1 tsp Ground turmeric

1/4 Juice of a lemon

For the spicy celery

1 tsp Extra virgin olive oil

40 g Red onion, finely chopped

60 g Tinned green lentils

1 Garlic clove, finely chopped

1 cm Fresh ginger, finely chopped

1 Bire's eye chilli, finely chopped

150 g Celery, cut into 2cm lengths

1 tsp Mild curry powder

130 g Tomato, cut into 8 wedges

100 ml Chicken or vegetable stock

1 tbsp Chopped parsley

Instructions

1. Heat the oven to 200C / gas mark 6.

2. Start with the spicy celery. Heat a frying pan over a medium–low heat, add the olive oil, then the onion, garlic, ginger, chilli and celery. Fry gently for 2–3 minutes or until softened but not coloured, then add the curry powder and cook for a further minute.

3. Add the tomatoes then the stock and lentils and simmer gently for 10 minutes. You may want to increase or decrease the cooking time depending on how crunchy you like your celery.

4. Meanwhile, mix the turmeric, oil and lemon juice and rub over the salmon. # Place on a baking tray and cook for 8–10 minutes.

5. To finish, stir the parsley through the celery and serve with the salmon.

CORONATION CHICKEN SALAD

Preparation time: 5 minutes

Serves 1

Ingredients

75 g Natural yoghurt

Juice of 1/4 of a lemon

1 tsp Coriander, chopped

1 tsp Ground turmeric

1/2 tsp Mild curry powder

100 g Cooked chicken breast, cut into bite-sized pieces

6 Walnut halves, finely chopped

1 Medjool date, finely chopped

20 g Red onion, diced

1 Bird's eye chilli

40 g Rocket, to serve

Instructions

Mix the yoghurt, lemon juice, coriander and spices together in a bowl. Add all the remaining ingredients and serve on a bed of the rocket.

GRAPE AND MELON JUICE-SIRTFOOD RECIPES

Prep Time: 2 mins

Serves 1

Ingredients

½ cucumber, peeled if preferred, halved, seeds removed and roughly chopped

30g young spinach leaves, stalks removed

100g red seedless grapes

100g cantaloupe melon, peeled, deseeded and cut into chunks

Instruction

Blend together in a juicer or blender until smooth.

BAKED POTATOES WITH SPICY CHICKPEA STEW

Prep Time: 10 mins

Cook Time: 1 hour

Serves 4-6

Ingredients

4-6 baking potatoes, pricked all over

2 tablespoons olive oil

2 red onions, finely chopped

4 cloves garlic, grated or crushed

2cm ginger, grated

½ -2 teaspoons chilli flakes (depending on how hot you like things)

2 tablespoons cumin seeds

2 tablespoons turmeric

Splash of water

2 x 400g tins chopped tomatoes

2 tablespoons unsweetened cocoa powder (or cacao)

2 x 400g tins chickpeas (or kidney beans if you prefer) including the chickpea water DON'T DRAIN!!

2 yellow peppers (or whatever colour you prefer!), chopped into bitesize pieces

2 tablespoons parsley plus extra for garnish

Salt and pepper to taste (optional)

Side salad (optional)

Instructions

1. Preheat the oven to 200C, meanwhile you can prepare all your ingredients.

2. When the oven is hot enough put your baking potatoes in the oven and cook for 1 hour or until they are done how you like them.

3. Once the potatoes are in the oven, place the olive oil and chopped red onion in a large wide saucepan and cook gently, with the lid on for 5 minutes, until the onions are soft but not brown.

4. Remove the lid and add the garlic, ginger, cumin and chilli. Cook for a further minute on a low heat, then add the turmeric and a very small splash of water and cook for another minute, taking care not to let the pan get too dry.

5. Next, add in the tomatoes, cocoa powder (or cacao), chickpeas (including the chickpea water) and yellow pepper. Bring to the boil, then simmer on a low heat for 45 minutes until the sauce is thick and unctuous (but don't let it burn!). The stew should be done at roughly the same time as the potatoes.

6. Finally stir in the 2 tablespoons of parsley, and some salt and pepper if you wish, and serve the stew on top of the baked potatoes, perhaps with a simple side salad.

KALE AND RED ONION DHAL WITH BUCKWHEAT

Prep Time: 5 mins

Cook Time: 25 mins

Serves 4

Ingredients

1 tablespoon olive oil

1 small red onion, sliced

3 garlic cloves, grated or crushed

2 cm ginger, grated

1 birds eye chilli, deseeded and finely chopped (more if you like things hot!)

2 teaspoons turmeric

2 teaspoons garam masala

160g red lentils

400ml coconut milk

200ml water

100g kale (or spinach would be a great alternative)

160g buckwheat (or brown rice)

Instructions

1. Put the olive oil in a large, deep saucepan and add the sliced onion. Cook on a low heat, with the lid on for 5 minutes until softened.

2. Add the garlic, ginger and chilli and cook for 1 more minute.

3. Add the turmeric, garam masala and a splash of water and cook for 1 more minute.

4. Add the red lentils, coconut milk, and 200ml water (do this simply by half filling the coconut milk can with water and tipping it into the saucepan).

5. Mix everything together thoroughly and cook for 20 minutes over a gently heat with the lid on. Stir occasionally and add a little more water if the dhal starts to stick.

6. After 20 minutes add the kale, stir thoroughly and replace the lid, cook for a further 5 minutes (1-2 minutes if you use spinach instead!)

7. About 15 minutes before the curry is ready, place the buckwheat in a medium saucepan and add plenty of boiling water. Bring the water back to the boil and cook for 10 minutes (or a little longer if you prefer your buckwheat softer. Drain the buckwheat in a sieve and serve with the dhal.

CHARGRILLED BEEF WITH A RED WINE JUS, ONION RINGS, GARLIC KALE AND HERB ROASTED POTATOES

Ingredients

100g potatoes, peeled and cut into 2cm dice

1 tbsp extra virgin olive oil

5g parsley, finely chopped

50g red onion, sliced into rings

50g kale, sliced

1 garlic clove, finely chopped

120–150g x 3.5cm-thick beef fillet steak or 2cm-thick sirloin steak

40ml red wine

150ml beef stock

1 tsp tomato purée

1 tsp cornflour, dissolved in 1 tbsp water

Instructions

1. Heat the oven to 220°C/gas 7.

2. Place the potatoes in a saucepan of boiling water, bring back to the boil and cook for 4–5 minutes, then drain. Place in a roasting tin with 1 teaspoon of the oil

and roast in the hot oven for 35–45 minutes. Turn the potatoes every 10 minutes to ensure even cooking. When cooked, remove from the oven, sprinkle with the chopped parsley and mix well.

3. Fry the onion in 1 teaspoon of the oil over a medium heat for 5–7 minutes, until soft and nicely caramelised. Keep warm. Steam the kale for 2–3 minutes then drain. Fry the garlic gently in ½ teaspoon of oil for 1 minute, until soft but not coloured. Add the kale and fry for a further 1–2 minutes, until tender. Keep warm.

4. Heat an ovenproof frying pan over a high heat until smoking. Coat the meat in ½ a teaspoon of the oil and fry in the hot pan over a medium–high heat according to how you like your meat done.If you like your meat medium it would be better to sear the meat and then transfer the pan to an oven set at 220°C/gas 7 and finish the cooking that way for the prescribed times.

5. Remove the meat from the pan and set aside to rest. Add the wine to the hot pan to bring up any meat residue. Bubble to reduce the wine by half, until syrupy and with a concentrated flavor.

6. Add the stock and tomato purée to the steak pan and bring to the boil, then add the cornflour paste to thicken your sauce, adding it a little at a time until you have your desired consistency. Stir in any of the juices from the rested steak and serve with the roasted potatoes, kale, onion rings and red wine sauce.

KALE AND BLACKCURRANT SMOOTHIE

Prep Time: 3 mins

Serves 2

Ingredeints

2 tsp honey

1 cup freshly made green tea

10 baby kale leaves, stalks removed

1 ripe banana

40 g blackcurrants, washed and stalks removed

6 ice cubes

Instruction

Stir the honey into the warm green tea until dissolved. Whiz all the ingredients together in a blender until smooth. Serve immediately.

BUCKWHEAT PASTA SALAD

Serves 1

Ingredients

50g buckwheat pasta(cooked according to the packet instructions)

large handful of rocket

small handful of basil leaves

8 cherry tomatoes,halved

1/2 avocado,diced

10 olives

1 tbsp extra virgin olive oil

20g pine nuts

Instruction

Gently combine all the ingredients except the pine nuts and arrange on a plate or in a bowl,then scatter the pine nuts over the top.

GREEK SALAD SKEWERS

Prep Time; 10mins

Serves 2

Ingredients

2 wooden skewers, soaked in water for 30 minutes before use

8 large black olives

8 cherry tomatoes

1 yellow pepper, cut into 8 squares

½ red onion, cut in half and separated into 8 pieces

100g (about 10cm) cucumber, cut into 4 slices and halved

100g feta, cut into 8 cubes

For the dressing:

1 tbsp extra virgin olive oil

Juice of ½ lemon

1 tsp balsamic vinegar

½ clove garlic, peeled and crushed

Few leaves basil, finely chopped (or ½ tsp dried mixed herbs to replace basil and oregano)

Few leaves oregano, finely chopped

Generous seasoning of salt and freshly ground black pepper

Instructions

1. Thread each skewer with the salad ingredients in the order: olive, tomato, yellow pepper, red onion, cucumber, feta, tomato, olive, yellow pepper, red onion, cucumber, feta.

2. Place all the dressing ingredients in a small bowl and mix together thoroughly. Pour over the skewers.

KALE, EDAMAME AND TOFU CURRY

Ready in 45 minutes

 Serves 4

Ingredients

1 tbsp rapeseed oil

1 large onion, chopped

4 cloves garlic, peeled and grated

1 large thumb (7cm) fresh ginger, peeled and grated

1 red chilli, deseeded and thinly sliced

1/2 tsp ground turmeric

1/4 tsp cayenne pepper

1 tsp paprika

1/2 tsp ground cumin

1 tsp salt

250g dried red lentils

1 litre boiling water

50g frozen soyaedamame beans

200g firm tofu, chopped into cubes

2 tomatoes, roughly chopped

Juice of 1 lime

200g kale leaves, stalks removed and torn

Instructions

1. Put the oil in a heavy-bottomed pan over a low-medium heat. Add the onion and cook for 5 minutes before adding the garlic, ginger and chilli and cooking for a further 2 minutes. Add the turmeric, cayenne, paprika, cumin and salt. Stir through before adding the red lentils and stirring again.

2. Pour in the boiling water and bring to a hearty simmer for 10 minutes, then reduce the heat and cook for a further 20-30 minutes until the curry has a thick '•porridge' consistency.

3. Add the soya beans, tofu and tomatoes and cook for a further 5 minutes. Add the lime juice and kale leaves and cook until the kale is just tender.

CHOCOLATE CUPCAKES WITH MATCHA ICING

Ready in 35 minutes

Servings 12

Ingredients

150g self-raising flour

200g caster sugar

60g cocoa

½ tsp salt

½ tsp fine espresso coffee, decaf if preferred

120ml milk

½ tsp vanilla extract

50ml vegetable oil

1 egg

120ml boiling water

For the icing:

50g butter, at room temperature

50g icing sugar

1 tbsp matcha green tea powder

½ tsp vanilla bean paste

50g soft cream cheese

Instructions

1. Preheat the oven to 180C/160C fan. Line a cupcake tin with paper or silicone cake cases.

2. Place the flour, sugar, cocoa, salt and espresso powder in a large bowl and mix thoroughly.

3. Add the milk, vanilla extract, vegetable oil and egg to the dry ingredients and use an electric mixer to beat until well combined. Carefully pour in the boiling water slowly and beat on a low speed until fully combined. Use a high speed to beat for a further minute to add air to the batter. The batter is much more liquid than a normal cake mix. Have faith, it will taste amazing!

4. Spoon the batter evenly between the cake cases. Each cake case should be no more than ¾ full. Bake in the oven for 15-18 minutes, until the mixture bounces back when tapped. Remove from the oven and allow to cool completely before icing.

5. To make the icing, cream the butter and icing sugar together until it's pale and smooth. Add the matcha powder and vanilla and stir again. Finally add the cream cheese and beat until smooth. Pipe or spread over the cakes.

SESAME CHICKEN SALAD

Ready in 12 minutes

Serves 2

Ingredients

1 tbsp sesame seeds

1 cucumber, peeled, halved lengthways, deseeded with a teaspoon and sliced

100g baby kale, roughly chopped

60g pak choi, very finely shredded

½ red onion, very finely sliced

Large handful (20g) parsley, chopped

150g cooked chicken, shredded

For the dressing:

1 tbsp extra virgin olive oil

1 tsp sesame oil

Juice of 1 lime

1 tsp clear honey

2 tsp soy sauce

Instructions

1. Toast the sesame seeds in a dry frying pan for 2 minutes until lightly browned and fragrant. Transfer to a plate to cool.

2. In a small bowl, mix together the olive oil, sesame oil, lime juice, honey and soy sauce to make the dressing.

3. Place the cucumber, kale, pak choi, red onion and parsley in a large bowl and gently mix together. Pour over the dressing and mix again.

4. Distribute the salad between two plates and top with the shredded chicken. Sprinkle over the sesame seeds just before serving.

AROMATIC CHICKEN BREAST WITH KALE, RED ONION, AND SALSA

Ingredients

120g skinless, boneless chicken breast

2 tsp ground turmeric

juice of ¼ lemon

1 tbsp extra virgin olive oil

50g kale, chopped

20g red onion, sliced

1 tsp chopped fresh ginger

50g buckwheat

Instructions

1. To make the salsa, remove the eye from the tomato and chop it very finely, taking care to keep as much of the liquid as possible. Mix with the chilli, capers, parsley and lemon juice. You could put everything in a blender but the end result is a little different.

2. Heat the oven to 220°C/gas 7. Marinate the chicken breast in 1 teaspoon of the turmeric, the lemon juice and a little oil. Leave for 5–10 minutes.

3. Heat an ovenproof frying pan until hot, then add the marinated chicken and cook for a minute or so on each side, until pale golden, then transfer to the oven (place on a baking tray if your pan isn't ovenproof) for 8–10

minutes or until cooked through. Remove from the oven, cover with foil and leave to rest for 5 minutes before serving.

4. Meanwhile, cook the kale in a steamer for 5 minutes. Fry the red onions and the ginger in a little oil, until soft but not coloured, then add the cooked kale and fry for another minute.

5. Cook the buckwheat according to the packet instructions with the remaining teaspoon of turmeric. Serve alongside the chicken, vegetables and salsa.

SMOKED SALMON OMELETTE

Prep Time: 5 – 10 minutes

Serves 1

Ingredients

2 Medium eggs

100 g Smoked salmon, sliced

1/2 tsp Capers

10 g Rocket, chopped

1 tsp Parsley, chopped

1 tsp Extra virgin olive oil

Instrctions

1. Crack the eggs into a bowl and whisk well. Add the salmon, capers, rocket and parsley.

2. Heat the olive oil in a non-stick frying pan until hot but not smoking. Add the egg mixture and, using a spatula or fish slice, move the mixture around the pan until it is even. Reduce the heat and let the omelette cook through. Slide the spatula around the edges and roll up or fold the omelette in half to serve.

GREEN TEA SMOOTHIE

Ready in 3 minutes

Serves 2

Ingredients

2 ripe bananas

250 ml milk

2 tsp matcha green tea powder

1/2 tsp vanilla bean paste (not extract) or a small scrape of the seeds from a vanilla pod

6 ice cubes

2 tsp honey

Instruction

1. Simply blend all the ingredients together in a blender and serve in two glasses.

SIRT FOOD MISO MARINATED COD WITH STIR FRIED GREENS & SESAME

Serves 1

Ingredients

20g miso

1 tbsp mirin

1 tbsp extra virgin olive oil

200g skinless cod fillet

20g red onion, sliced

40g celery, sliced

1 garlic clove, finely chopped

1 bird's eye chilli, finely chopped

1 tsp finely chopped fresh ginger

60g green beans

50g kale, roughly chopped

1 tsp sesame seeds

5g parsley, roughly chopped

1 tbsp tamari

30g buckwheat

1 tsp ground turmeric

Instructions

1. Mix the miso, mirin and 1 teaspoon of the oil. Rub all over the cod and leave to marinate for 30 minutes. Heat the oven to 220°C/gas 7.

2. Bake the cod for 10 minutes.

3. Meanwhile, heat a large frying pan or wok with the remaining oil. Add the onion and stir-fry for a few minutes, then add the celery, garlic, chilli, ginger, green beans and kale. Toss and fry until the kale is tender and cooked through. You may need to add a little water to the pan to aid the cooking process.

4. Cook the buckwheat according to the packet instructions with the turmeric for 3 minutes.

5. Add the sesame seeds, parsley and tamari to the stir-fry and serve with the greens and fish.

APPLE PANCAKES WITH BLACKCURRANT COMPOTE

Ready in 20 minutes

Serves 4

Ingredients

75g porridge oats

125g plain flour

1 tsp baking powder

2 tbsp caster sugar

Pinch of salt

2 apples, peeled, cored and cut into small pieces

300ml semi-skimmed milk

2 egg whites

2 tsp light olive oil

For the compote:

120g blackcurrants, washed and stalks removed

2 tbsp caster sugar

3 tbsp water

Instructions

1. First make the compote. Place the blackcurrants, sugar and water in a small pan. Bring up to a simmer and cook for 10-15 minutes.

2. Place the oats, flour, baking powder, caster sugar and salt in a large bowl and mix well. Stir in the apple and then whisk in the milk a little at a time until you have a smooth mixture. Whisk the egg whites to stiff peaks and then fold into the pancake batter. Transfer the batter to a jug.

3. Heat 1/2 tsp oil in a non-stick frying pan on a medium-high heat and pour in approximately one quarter of the batter. Cook on both sides until golden brown. Remove and repeat to make four pancakes.

4. Serve the pancakes with the blackcurrant compote drizzled over.

SIRT FRUIT SALAD

Ready in 10 minutes

Serves 1

Ingredients

½ cup freshly made green tea

1 tsp honey

1 orange, halved

1 apple, cored and roughly chopped

10 red seedless grapes

10 blueberries

Instructions

1. Stir the honey into half a cup of green tea. When dissolved, add the juice of half the orange. Leave to cool.

2. Chop the other half of the orange and place in a bowl together with the chopped apple, grapes and blueberries. Pour over the cooled tea and leave to steep for a few minutes before serving.

SIRT MUESLI

Ingredients

20g buckwheat flakessirtfood recipes

10g buckwheat puffs

15g coconut flakes or desiccated coconut

40g Medjool dates, pitted and chopped

15g walnuts, chopped

10g cocoa nibs

100g strawberries, hulled and chopped

100g plain Greek yoghurt (or vegan alternative, such as soya or coconut yoghurt)

Instructions

Mix all of the above ingredients together, only adding the yoghurt and strawberries before serving if you are making it in bulk.

SIRTFOOD BITES

Ingredients

120g walnuts

30g dark chocolate (85 per cent cocoa solids), broken into pieces; or cocoa nibs

250g Medjool dates, pitted

1 tbsp cocoa powder

1 tbsp ground turmeric

1 tbsp extra virgin olive oil

the scraped seeds of one vanilla pod or 1 tsp vanilla extract

1–2 tbsp water

Instructions

1. Place the walnuts and chocolate in a food processor and process until you have a fine powder.

2. Add all the other ingredients except the water and blend until the mixture forms a ball. You may or may not have to add the water depending on the consistency of the mixture – you don't want it to be too sticky.

3. Using your hands, form the mixture into bite-sized balls and refrigerate in an airtight container for at least one hour before eating them.

4. You could roll some of the balls in some more cocoa or desiccated coconut to achieve a different finish if you like.

5. They will keep for up to one week in your fridge.

CHINESE-STYLE PORK WITH PAK CHOI

Serves 4

Ingredients

400g firm tofu, cut into large cubes

1 tbsp cornfloursirtfood recipes

1 tbsp water

125ml chicken stock

1 tbsp rice wine

1 tbsp tomato pure´e

1 tsp brown sugar

1 tbsp soy sauce

1 clove garlic, peeled and crushed

1 thumb (5cm) fresh ginger, peeled and grated 1 tbsp rapeseed oil

100g shiitake mushrooms, sliced

1 shallot, peeled and sliced

200g pak choi or choi sum, cut into thin slices 400g pork mince (10% fat)

100g beansprouts

Large handful (20g) parsley, chopped

Instructions

1. Lay out the tofu on kitchen paper, cover with more kitchen paper and set aside.

2. In a small bowl, mix together the cornflour and water, removing all lumps. Add the chicken stock, rice wine, tomato pure´e, brown sugar and soy sauce. Add the crushed garlic and ginger and stir together.

3. In a wok or large frying pan, heat the oil to a high temperature. Add the shiitake mushrooms and stir-fry for 2–3 minutes until cooked and glossy. Remove the mushrooms from the pan with a slotted spoon and set aside. Add the tofu to the pan and stir-fry until golden on all sides. Remove with a slotted spoon and set aside.

4. Add the shallot and pak choi to the wok, stir-fry for 2 minutes, then add the mince. Cook until the mince is cooked through, then add the sauce, reduce the heat a notch and allow the sauce to bubble round the meat for a minute or two. Add the beansprouts, shiitake mushrooms and tofu to the pan and warm through. Remove from the heat, stir through the parsley and serve immediately.

TUSCAN BEAN STEW-SIRTFOOD RECIPES

Ingredients

1 tbsp extra virgin olive oil

50g red onion, finely chopped

30g carrot, peeled and finely choppedsirtfood recipes

30g celery, trimmed and finely chopped

1 garlic clove, finely chopped

½ bird's eye chilli, finely chopped (optional)

1 tsp herbes de Provence

200ml vegetable stock

1 x 400g tin chopped Italian tomatoes

1 tsp tomato purée

200g tinned mixed beans

50g kale, roughly chopped

1 tbsp roughly chopped parsley

40g buckwheat

Instructions

1. Place the oil in a medium saucepan over a low–medium heat and gently fry the onion, carrot, celery, garlic, chilli(if using) and herbs, until the onion is soft but not colored.

2. Add the stock, tomatoes and tomato purée and bring to the boil. Add the beans and simmer for 30 minutes.

3. Add the kale and cook for another 5–10 minutes, until tender, then add the parsley.

4. Meanwhile, cook the buckwheat according to the packet instructions, drain and then serve with the stew.

SALMON SIRT SUPER SALAD

Servings 1

Ingredients

50g rocket

50g chicory leaves

100g smoked salmon slices (you can also use lentils, cooked chicken breast or tinned tuna)

80g avocado, peeled, stoned and sliced

40g celery, sliced

20g red onion, sliced

15g walnuts, chopped

1 tbs capers

1 large Medjool date, pitted and chopped

1 tbs extra-virgin olive oil

Juice ¼ lemon

10g parsley, chopped

10g lovage or celery leaves, chopped

Instructions

Arrange the salad leaves on a large plate. Mix all the remaining ingredients together and serve on top of the leaves.

A 21-DAY SIRTFOOD DIET PLAN

Week One	8 a.m.	12 p.m.	4 p.m.	8 p.m.
Monday	Grape and Melon Juice	Kale and Blackcurrant Smoothie	Green Tea Smoothie	Tumeric Chicken Salad with honey lime dressing
Tuesday	Sirtfood Green Juice	Sirt Muesli	Sirt fruit Salad	Buckwheat noodles with Chicken kale and Miso Dressing
Wednesday	Green Tea Smoothie	Grape and Melon Juice	Kale and Blackcurrant Smoothie	Asian King Prawn Stir-Fry with Buckwheat Noodles
Thursday	Sirt fruit Salad	Sirtfood Green Juice	Sirt Muesli	Baked Salad with Creamy Mind Dressing
Friday	Kale Blackcurrant Smoothie	Green Tea Smoothie	Grape and Melon Smoothie	Chic Chip Granola
Saturday	Sirt Muesli	Sirt fruit Salad	Sirtfood Green Juice	Fragrant Asian Hotspot
Sunday	Grape and Melon Juice	Kale and Blackcurrant Smoothie	Green Tea Smoothie	Lamb, Butternut Squash and Date Tagine

	8 a.m.	12 p.m.	4 p.m.	8 p.m.
Week Two				
Monday	Kale and Blackcurrant Smoothie	Sirtfood Green Juice	Greek Salad Skewers	Prawn Arrabbiata
Tuesday	Sirt fruit Salad	Green Tea Smoothie	Kale, Edamame and Tofu curry	Tumeric baked Salmon
Wednesday	Green Tea Smoothie	Grape and Melon Smoothie	Sesame Chicken Salad	Coronation Chicken Salad
Thursday	Sirtfood Green Juice	Sirt Muesli	Sirtfood Mushroom Scramble Eggs	Baked Potatoes with Spicy Chickpea Stew
Friday	Grape and Melon Juice	Kale and Blackcurrant Smoothie	Aromatic Chicken Breast With Kale, Red onions...	Kale and Red Onion Dhal with Buckwheat
Saturday	Sirt Muesli	Sirt fruit Salad	Smoked Salmon Omelette	Chargrilled Beef with Red wine.
Sunday	Kale and Blackcurrant Smoothie	Green Tea Smoothie	Sirtfood Miso Marinated with Sirtfood greens and Semame	Buckwheat Pasta Salad

Week Three	8 a.m.	12 p.m.	4 p.m.	8 p.m.
Monday	Salmon Sirt Super Salad	Fragrant Asian Hotspot	Raspberry and Blackcurrant Jelly	Grape and Melon Juice
Tuesday	Prawn Arrabbiata	Lamb and Butternut Squash and Date Tagine	Apple Pancakes with Blackcurrant Compote	Kale and Blackcurrant Smoothie
Wednesday	Buckwheat Pasta Salad	Choc Chip Granola	Sirtfood bites	Kale, Edamame and Tofu curry
Thursday	Tumeric baked Salmon	Baked Salad with Creamy Mint Dressing	Chinese-style Pork with Pak Choi	Green tea smoothie
Friday	Sirtfood bites	Smoked Salmon Omelette	Tuscan Bean Stew-sirtfood Reciipes	Sirt Fruit Salad
Saturday	Salmon Sirt Super Salad	Aromatic Chicken Breast with Kale, Red onions...	Salmon Sirt Super Salad	Sirt food Green Juice
Sunday	Buckwheat Noodles	Shrimp Stir-fry	Miso-glazed Tofu	Sirt Muesli

CPSIA information can be obtained
at www.ICGtesting.com
Printed in the USA
BVHW061316310821
615692BV00003BA/259